SPIT THAT OUT!

Praise for *Spit That Out!*

A realistic guide to keeping your kids safe and healthy.

— *people.com*

New mom and healthy living advocate Paige Wolf provides truths, tips, and mom-to-mom advice on how to go green without going insane in this humorous must-read.

— *Pregnancy & Newborn Magazine*

Parents may be the guiltiest demographic, but [Wolf's] advice pertains to all those suffering a crisis of environmental conscience.

— *The Huffington Post*

...a must read for eco-concerned parents.

— *babble.com*

For a book about all the mom-things that have been stressing me out, *Spit That Out!* actually de-stressed me. Paige gives simple, reasonable, 'you don't have to do it all' suggestions, which make me feel like a slightly less horrible mother.

— Vicki Glembocki, author of *The Second Nine Months: One Woman Tells the Real Truth About Becoming a Mom. Finally.*

Paige Wolf is the mom I wished lived next door. She makes neurotic look sexy and shares practical tips for saving the ozone and your sanity.

— Abby Sher, author of *Amen, Amen, Amen: Memoir of a Girl Who Couldn't Stop Praying (Among Other Things)*

Creating an eco-healthy life has a learning curve, and it's great to know someone has the answers when I need them.

— Angie Goff, NBC Washington News Anchor

Wolf offers practical suggestions for both managing your house and managing your emotions when you feel overwhelmed.

— *apartmenttherapy.com*

Plenty of good tips on maintaining our sanity in a world where we're supposed to keep track of our impact in every possible direction.

— *Philadelphia Daily News*

Spit That Out! reads fast, fun and focused. It's as if you had a non-judgmental new mom group right there between the covers as your touchstone, giving each mom the support and information to make the decision that's best for her family. How refreshing is that?

— *Cool Mom Picks*

SPIT THAT OUT!

The Overly Informed Parent's Guide to Raising
Healthy Kids in the Age of Environmental Guilt

Paige Wolf

Foreword by **Alysia Reiner**

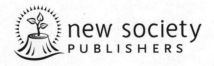

new society
PUBLISHERS

Cover design by Diane McIntosh. Image © iStock.
Interior images © Adobe Stock: NokHoOkNoi, Natis, Séa,
d'Naya, BF Grafik, John Takai, hermandesign2015, Jane.

Printed in Canada. First printing September 2016.

Funded by the	Financé par le	
Government	gouvernement	**Canadä**
of Canada	du Canada	

Inquiries regarding requests to reprint all or part of *Spit That Out!* should be addressed to New Society Publishers at the address below. To order directly from the publishers, please call toll-free (North America) 1-800-567-6772, or order online at www.newsociety.com.

Any other inquiries can be directed by mail to:

New Society Publishers
P.O. Box 189, Gabriola Island, BC V0R 1X0, Canada
(250) 247-9737

LIBRARY AND ARCHIVES CANADA CATALOGUING IN PUBLICATION

Wolf, Paige, author
Spit that out! : the overly informed parent's guide to raising healthy kids in the age of environmental guilt / Paige Wolf ; foreword by Alysia Reiner.

Includes bibliographical references and index.
Issued also in print and electronic formats.
ISBN 978-0-86571-830-2 (paperback). — ISBN 978-1-55092-625-5 (ebook)

1. Child rearing—Environmental aspects. 2. Parenting—
Environmental aspects. 3. Green movement. 4. Sustainable living. I. Title.

| GE195.W65 2016 | 649'.1 | C2016-902759-7 |
| | | C2016-902760-0 |

New Society Publishers' mission is to publish books that contribute in fundamental ways to building an ecologically sustainable and just society, and to do so with the least possible impact on the environment, in a manner that models this vision. We are committed to doing this not just through education, but through action. The interior pages of our bound books are printed on Forest Stewardship Council®-registered acid-free paper that is 100% post-consumer recycled (100% old growth forest-free), processed chlorine-free, and printed with vegetable-based, low-VOC inks, with covers produced using FSC®-registered stock. New Society also works to reduce its carbon footprint, and purchases carbon offsets based on an annual audit to ensure a carbon neutral footprint. For further information, or to browse our full list of books and purchase securely, visit our website at: www.newsociety.com.

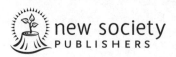

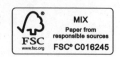

To my children, Sam and Evelyn,
who keep me constantly on edge and in awe.

Contents

I did then what I knew how to do.
Now that I know better, I do better.

— Maya Angelou

Foreword

by Alysia Reiner

This summer my daughter looked at the sprinkles on her ice cream and asked what was in them. It was a one of those challenging (read: deeply sad/panic/green-guilt) moments.

I tend to play the 90/10 game: 90 percent of the time, at home and when I can, we go super healthy. I try to keep as many chemicals, artificial colors, flavors, preservatives, GMOs, hydrogenated oils, high-fructose corn syrups, etc. as I can out of our world. We do stuff like give away all our candy for Halloween, and she picks something from the Natural Candy Store instead. But I also try to not give her a complex about it. I don't want her to alienate or offend other people or their choices, and want her to feel unlimited in her world. So 10 percent of the time I say F*#$ it—everything in moderation, right?

So when she asked me the sprinkle question, I just wanted to hide under the covers. Sprinkles were a 10 percent area. I so didn't want to burst the bubble of joy all kids have about those multicolored fireworks that make ice cream super special.

Instead I told the truth. I didn't want to, and I told her that first: I didn't want to answer because it might ruin sprinkles for her. But she asked me to tell her anyway, so I talked about hydrogenated oils in a way a six-year-old can understand: what they do to your body (artificial colors and flavors she already knew about). And then I offered the option of looking for a healthy version. We found organic sprinkles made with natural colors, no oil, still yummy, and she still insists they taste better and the colors are prettier. We brought them with us when we went out for ice cream all summer, and it is now a lifelong habit and worth the carbon footprint of flying them to us in Fire Island.

Why You Should Buy and Read This Book: From my Seven-Year-Old Daughter

[Full disclosure: she did not read the book, but we kind of live it because I am a bit of a green neurotic.]

66 *I suggest you buy and read this book because I think it will help you a lot with you and your children. A lot of the things that this book tells you are not on any of the labels of any of the things you buy. I think this will make parenting easier because you do not have to worry about the things you or your child uses. I was raised this way, and once you start, there is no going back. You know what choices you want to make, and you can tell if something is natural or unnatural by heart.* 99

I think that says it all, right? Who needs me? What I can say is, truthy truth: she did grow up this way, and she does make amazing choices even when I am not around, which is the real test.

The other truth I have found is that in our current world, as evidenced above, there are so many amazing alternatives that are so much healthier for you, your kids, and the environment. And to reference the first chapter—those choices just weren't as readily available when we were kids.

So are you a good-news-first or a bad-news-first kind of person?

Me, I'm a bad-news-first gal, so that's how I will start this book. If you are a good-news-first human, skip to the big block letters below that say THE GOOD NEWS!

If not, let's start with a truth: parenting is super crazy scary! Learning you're pregnant—though hopefully a joy—is totally terrifying as well. Being responsible for the life of another human, keeping it alive and as healthy as possible, is no small task in our current world.

My first night with my daughter (after a super-easy, 100-percent natural birth at a birthing center where they kicked us out after 14 hours because it *was* so fast and free of complications) my husband

and I *both* hallucinated that it was 50 degrees Fahrenheit (we had turned the heat up to 80—it was *in fact, no joke*, 80 degrees in our bedroom) and our baby would freeze to death. I so wish I were kidding right now.

Oh and then there is that environmental and global warming thing that may make it so there will be no world for your kids to live in.

"More than 80,000 chemicals currently used in the US haven't been adequately tested for their effects on human health."
— Natural Resources Defense Council (NRDC)[1]

According to the World Health Organization, more than 50 percent of the one million annual child deaths from acute respiratory infections are attributable to indoor air pollution; acute poisoning from pesticides can be life-threatening to children, *and*, globally, 19 percent of all cancers are attributed to environmental factors, resulting in 1.3 million deaths each year.[2]

Even Bill Gates (kinda sorta really smart dude you may have heard of) believes if we don't start thinking about the environment more, there simply *won't be one for our kids*.[3]

You can spend *a lifetime* Googling and either:

a) Be more confused about what is good and bad for you and the world

Or

b) Feel so insanely guilty that you are not doing everything perfectly that you just want to hide your whole family in a sterile, chemical-free bubble. Well that, or go pour yourself a very dry organic fair-trade local martini with a twist from a lemon grown in your backyard.

I promise this book is the good news and part of the solution.

The Good News

We have all wished for a parenting handbook on a variety of topics in, well, eco-cool parenting—and now there is! And not only that, it isn't another "sancta-mommy" version of it all (we all know those sanctimonious books—and let's be honest, those *people*—who are all, "I know how to parent and you don't, so I will talk really slow til you understand how dumb you are.") Paige has a sense of *humor* and irony and, *thank you god*, she has been there, my friends. She gets it, and she is willing to tell her sprinkle stories.

And for that I am really thrilled and grateful to call her friend, and say, read this book.

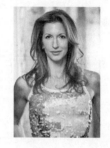

Actress, producer, and consummate Pollyanna, ALYSIA REINER uses her superpowers for good (even though she's known for playing some amazing bitches!). Alysia won her second SAG award for her role as Fig on "Orange is the New Black." She produced and starred in the movie *Equity*, the first female-driven Wall Street film, and is also known for her television work on "How to Get Away with Murder," "Rosewood," and "Better Things."

Preface

You are a great parent.

If you weren't, you wouldn't even worry about these things. You wouldn't think twice about what's in your child's cereal. Or think that you *should* be thinking about what's in your child's cereal.

Just the fact that this title spoke to you in any way means you care. You are ahead of the curve because you want to do better. You may even want to be perfect—but you can't be. No book will ever teach you that.

Perfect is unattainable.

But better is always possible.

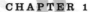

CHAPTER 1

Did What Our Parents Never Knew Hurt Us?

Navigating the New Normal

WHEN I WAS PREGNANT, I made one promise to myself. I would not be like my parents.

Neurotic to the core, they wanted to rush me to the emergency room every time I coughed, sure I was choking on a chicken bone (even though I'm pretty sure no one has ever found a bone in a McNugget).

I was going to let my children get scrapes on their knees and sneeze without fear of alarming their parents. I wasn't going to panic over a runny nose or sitting too close to the television.

And I was right. I am nothing like my parents. Because my special breed of neurosis is unique to the generation of climate change, consumer recalls, and information overload.

My hypochondria lies less in the here and now and more in whether my decisions will increase the likelihood of cancer in my children decades down the road. And if the Facebook groups, message boards, online forums, and chat rooms are any indication, many mothers in the 21st century are racked with environmental guilt, confusion, and panic.

In addition to the age-old, daunting task of raising a happy, healthy baby, we are bombarded with new and contradictory research concerning environmental toxins, long-term product effects, and the far-reaching impact of every item we purchase and decision we make. We want the world to be a better place not just for our children, but for the planet, which seems to be in dire peril.

Never has a generation been so inundated with conflicting information. We are the internet generation, and saying "what we don't know won't hurt us" is no longer an option when the answers are at our fingertips.

Most parents just want to do right by their children and society. We want to leave the world a better place and raise a better generation. We know that our voices count, and we are voting with everything we purchase, eat, and wear.

And with all this knowledge, we feel like we have no excuse for making the wrong decision. In the unachievable quest for parental perfection, all this information can be too much burden to carry.

Over the past five years, I've used my blog and social media to engage readers and experts, answering your questions on everything from leaching plastics to safer sunscreens to K-Cup addiction. On a quest to make green living more practical, manageable, and affordable, I searched high and low for the best hacks, bargains, and shortcuts to sort through the noise and find solutions that work. At the same time, health activists, dedicated brands, and a few forward-thinking policymakers have created significant progress. We've seen a consumer petition sway Kraft to remove artificial preservatives and dyes, various for-profit organizations offer rewards for recycling, and organizations gain national publicity for lobbying against the waste of misshapen tomatoes.[1]

But for every step forward, we often take two steps back, second-guessing our choices or just feeling too overwhelmed to care.

Sadly, it's pretty understandable when a family on a limited budget living in a "food desert" buys soda in bulk and embraces the McDonald's Dollar Menu.

But even some families armed with information and access appear oblivious when it comes to better food and product choices.

Why are well-meaning parents who pore over preschool options and violin lessons still making Cheez-Its—which use a chemical for "freshness" that the Toxicology Data Network links to chronic neuro-toxic effects—the default snack?[2] Why is sugar-laden Gatorade a reasonable beverage option for toddlers and artificially flavored Munchkin donut holes still the preferred school birthday snack? Why does my son keep asking me for bubble gum and feeling like the only one who can't go to the Mister Softee truck?

Joellen, a 38-year-old working mother of two in Moorestown, NJ, talks to me about why these things are still on her shopping list.

❝ *Sometimes I get caught up in this mindset that there are so many environmental dangers, why bother doing this because in the end, it's not going to make a difference?* ❞

But Joellen says the biggest problem is feeling like she only has the ability to worry about a certain number of things—she just doesn't have the capacity to add this to her guilt.

❝ *I feel like it has taken up all of my energy and time worrying about and controlling so many other things in my children's lives—making sure they're not getting too much screen time, making sure they're getting enough exercise, making sure I'm reading to them at night and practicing their numbers and letters.* ❞

Liz, a Philadelphia mother of two, offers the same sentiment of incapacitating panic.

❝ *I am worried about the chemicals in 'dollar store Barbie' and wonder if I should be more concerned. But then I forget about it because life is crazy and I don't have time to worry about every possible danger. Did I brush their teeth this morning? Are they eating healthy, balanced meals? Did I wash my hands before I pumped this milk? Did I pay attention to them equally? You could go crazy. Thank god for Zoloft, although I worry about taking worry medication!* ❞

Meghan, a mom in Mentor, OH, is equally overwhelmed.

> 66 *I feel like I'm constantly making lists on my phone of things to avoid or new brands to try out. I try to pay attention, stay informed, read labels, and research, but I am not always successful at that. Sometimes, I just want a bowl of Rice Krispies.* 99

These mothers' feelings of being overwhelmed make perfect sense. I can certainly understand the limited bandwidth for guilt.

A few years ago I cut out cow's milk as a way to decrease congestion. I discovered almond milk as an alternative and started using more than a gallon a week—in my oatmeal, my coffee, my protein shakes, my homemade ice cream.

But in the midst of California's historic drought, some have called for a boycott of my beloved almond milk. Eighty percent of the world's almond supply comes from that one state, where it takes 1.1 gallons of water to grow a single nut.[3]

Despite that knowledge, giving up almond milk has been beyond my personal capabilities for environmental good.

Bandwidth aside, Joellen also says she hasn't taken the time to really educate and inform herself.

> 66 *I feel like there's a lot of information out there, and I need to get the right information. I have a general sense of awareness from the media, but I don't want to jump on any bandwagon before I do the research myself—which is on my to-do list.* 99

Joellen says she needs to feel like it isn't being "shoved down her throat by someone else" and wants to take the time to educate herself about the real difference between two products.

> 66 *Why haven't I taken the time to educate myself? Do I really want to open that Pandora's box? Do I really want to start to know what I am exposed to? Because, then, how do I sleep at night? I just can't add that additional layer of stress and pressure on my life.* 99

But Joellen also acknowledges that she has only allowed herself to live in blissful ignorance because she hasn't had to deal with any visible effects from the traditional supermarket lifestyle.

❝ *I've been fortunate that in the microcosm of my life, my kids don't have any significant allergies or health problems. So I've never had to do that self-examination, like, 'Is there something I'm doing that's causing this?'* **❞**

Another somewhat surprising realization from my talk with parents has been their admissions of "blind product loyalty," perhaps a leftover hallmark of the Pepsi generation. Joellen says she doesn't know if an organic brand of chocolate sandwich cookies would taste the same. She says her kids would notice a subtle difference, and even she will miss the pleasure of that familiar taste.

It sounds like the true impetus to change is familiarity, as her kids have completely embraced Annie's Organic Cheddar Bunnies as an alternative to Goldfish. Why? Because they see other kids eating Cheddar Bunnies. They *know* Cheddar Bunnies.

But if she sees Cheerios right next to Cascadian Farm Organic O's for the same price, which will she buy?

❝ *Cheerios.* **❞**

We can probably all relate to brand loyalty on some level. My personal brand loyalty has been to Heinz Ketchup, as no other ketchup tastes quite right to me. Fortunately, the brand now offers an organic variety, which I am willing to pay a bit more for. (They also offer a third option called Simply Heinz, which uses real sugar in lieu of high-fructose corn syrup. I am continually curious why Simply Heinz isn't just, you know, Heinz.)

Ryan, a father of two, also confesses an ingrained trust in the brands he knew as a child.

❝ *We buy things we see in commercials not even thinking about it because we instinctively trust the brands. We see the same boxes from our childhood and don't consider that the ingredients or manufacturing process may have changed.* **❞**

But once things hit mainstream news, it can be a scary wake-up call.

❝ *We always saw Purdue as a trusted family brand, but then we saw some TV exposé about what's really going on at these poultry factory farms—it's not the same as 50 years ago. When we saw that, we started buying organic chicken.* ❞

For parents like Joellen, brand loyalty extends to the general comfort zone we were raised in—like the definition of "clean." Our parents found solace in the crisp, cool blue of a window cleaner bottle, rather than feeling like they were punched in the face by ammonia.

❝ *I tried a green cleaning service with DIY products and just felt like it wasn't working. The surfaces didn't feel the same.* ❞

While she recognizes her preconceived notion of "clean" is misguided, it's also a long way to go from bleach to vinegar. There are plenty of happy mediums along the way, and Joellen feels like she's finally ready to start taking the small steps.

❝ *If I can just start with the things that my family uses the most, I can get the most bang for my buck.* ❞

My hope is that this book will give you the tools to get that bang for your buck—financially, emotionally, and environmentally. We can lift the crushing weight off our shoulders and arm ourselves with bite-size pieces of information to increase our positive impact and our imprint.

Robyn O'Brien, a former food industry analyst, author of *The Unhealthy Truth*, and founder of the AllergyKids Foundation, is a calming yet commanding voice in the sea change.

❝ *You can look at all of this startling information and it feels like a tsunami coming at you and you experience total paralysis. But then I look at the four kids in my backyard and think, 'I can't not do something.'* ❞

One parent alone cannot hold back a tsunami, but we can form a thunderclap. And these thunderclaps are happening in corporate boardrooms, on the congressional floor, and in the nation's playgrounds.

This book will show you how parents can take on behemoth corporations, city councils, school districts, and their own opinionated 3rd graders—and win. We can't do everything, but we *can do something*. And we are exponentially stronger together.

CHAPTER 2

Can an Apple a Day Keep the Fast Food Mascots Away?

Managing a Clean, Green Family Diet

I USED TO BE A SUCKER for a sparkly Granny Smith—until I learned what gave apples their shine. Then I joined much of the nation in its embrace of all things organic, learning not to judge a fruit by its cover. Even if it sometimes looks a bit worse for the wear, the truth is that organic food usually *tastes* better.

It's easy to embrace fresh, sustainable produce when you can find and afford it. In fact, popular activists like Michael Pollen advocate a plant-based diet, and movies like *Food, Inc.*, *Fed Up*, and *Fast Food Nation* are enough to give anyone pause about their next Big Mac.

When our children are babies, we can protect them from less than perfect food. Those Golden Arches mean nothing to them, and we can raise them on nothing but breast milk and strained organic peas.

But then, when they are toddlers, you go to the playground and someone offers him a Goldfish, the unofficial universal snack, "made with smiles"—and MSG (labeled as autolyzed yeast) and very likely GMOs (conventional canola and soybean oils are almost assuredly made from genetically modified crops).

Goldfish feel to me like a gateway drug to toddler junk food. Soon, they are discovering bubble gum and lollipops, a rainbow dropping from the piñata at every child's birthday party.

We don't want to force them to live in a bubble, but we are a little freaked out to learn that vending machine-style peanut butter crackers are the daily snack at daycare.

Vicki Glembocki, author of *The Second Nine Months*, says when she was pregnant, she swore her kids would never eat fast food. But since she's become a mother she's realized, "you don't know what you don't know."

❝ It's not like we eat at Taco Bell three times a week or anything, but when there are starving, whining, screaming kids in the car, I believe that a Happy Meal is exactly that…a happy-making meal. ❞

Amy Wilson, actress and author of *When Did I Get Like This?*, says that, as with most parenting, there is a real continuum on the healthy eating scale.

❝ I have a friend who feeds her children much better than I ever have, or could. But we both have another friend who feeds her kids sugary cereals and artificial chocolate drinks for breakfast. I'm not as health-conscious as the one but not quite as vending machine as the other, and I can at least feel good about that. ❞

Actress Alysia Reiner ("Orange is the New Black") aims to feed her daughter organic but also understands the reality of living in an imperfect world.

❝ At home, I make organic pancakes and use local maple syrup. And then my husband takes my daughter Liv to the deli around the corner. Liv knows the name of the guy in the deli, and he always makes her these little pancakes. They use lard and corn syrup with artificial colors. It's so hard because that interaction with the man at the deli is a beautiful experience. She's learning about life and the world, and I don't want to say, 'You can't eat that!' ❞

Amy Wilson says when she is up against a culinary dilemma, she tries to get her three children involved in the food choices they make.

❝ I got rid of my kids' favorite breakfast cereal, Cinnamon Life, once I read the label and discovered it has artificial red and blue coloring in it. 'Why?' I ask you. Cinnamon Life is brown. The kids were disappointed. I explained that I was disappointed too, but I wasn't going to give them something that I was pretty sure was bad for them, and that we could find lots of cereals that weren't made that way. They accepted that explanation more readily than I would ever have expected, and they don't even ask for Cinnamon Life anymore. ❞

And then, of course, there is the ice cream truck, parents' enemy No. 1.

Dani Klein, comedian and author of *Afterbirth: Stories You Won't Read in a Parenting Magazine*, says Mister Softee falls into her "rage du jour" category.

❝ Every time I see that guy I feel my blood boil. And he shows up exactly when he knows the bus is going to pull up. I hate that they put parents in the position of having to say no. I tried to tell him once, but he was not receptive to my rant. I called the school too. Nothing. It's a free country. Honestly, I think they should be outlawed around schools! ❞

Michele Beschen, host of *b. organic with Michele Beschen* on PBS, is known for her do-it-yourself approach to green living. But she says despite raising her children with an avid emphasis on homegrown, wholesome food, her family has not gone without a fast-food fight.

In particular, Michele points to an ongoing battle over Kraft Lunchables—strategically packaged bite-size portions of deli meats, cheese, and crackers (along with candies like Airheads and Nerds) that I remember pining for in elementary school.

❝ My daughter would look longingly at that aisle every time we'd grocery shop, and you'd think I was denying her one of the greatest things on earth. I would even try to have fun creating our own healthier *versions of these compartmentalized, kid-mesmerizing foods. They just weren't as exciting to her, so I admit I have broken down and once in a great while, she gets to have one. The frequency of the requests has dwindled, and I do believe the novelty is tiring. Hopefully that means her taste buds are naturally becoming more in tune with better things.* **99**

Dawn Lerman, author of *My Fat Dad: A Memoir of Food, Love and Family, with Recipes*, says she is able to avoid "snack envy" by always being equipped.

66 *Once a week I make a big batch of cookies or brownies that look the same but are made with super healthy ingredients. But if they are at a party I let them eat whatever they want—I just try to feed them before-hand so they're not super hungry.* **99**

Robyn O'Brien believes natural foods shouldn't have to come at a premium or be snuck into parties. They should be the rule, not the exception.

66 *Organic is such a loaded term, but it's simply an adjective that describes the way a food is grown. Our grandparents didn't need that adjective—they just called it food.* **99**

But despite the Kool-Aid Man mascot still being a hit at the Macy's Thanksgiving Day Parade, Americans do realize there's something very wrong with our food system. And we're starting to speak up.

The cultural shift toward environmental and health awareness occurred so quickly that members of the mainstream food industry found themselves in a dilemma.

Big Food (America's top 25 food companies) has seen its market share dropping. Since 2005, children's cereal sales have fallen 10.7 percent[1] and canned soup sales have dropped 13 percent.[2] The first quarter of 2015 was the third consecutive quarter of declining sales and the fifth quarter of profit falls for McDonald's.[3]

Big box stores like Target and Walmart began rearranging their shelves so that major prepackaged foods with mascot branding were no longer at the lucrative eye level.

People are waking up.

And with that, Big Food had a couple choices: give the new, savvier consumers what they want or try to win back public perception.

Let's start with the latter.

Just as parents began uncovering the truth about pesticides, artificial dyes, and GMOs, the backlash began.

Some people claim that shopping organic is pointless or even pretentious. They call concerned shoppers "alarmists," and suddenly we second-guess ourselves, questioning whether it's worth spending that extra dollar for organic apples.

In May 2014, New York parents were invited to attend an event titled "From Helicopter to Hazmat: How the Culture of Alarmism Is Turning Parenting Into a Dangerous Job," presented by Independent Women's Forum (IWF). IWF is a conservative nonprofit organization whose key efforts include advocating against certain manufacturing safeguards and government regulations pertaining to the use of potentially toxic chemicals. They believe "radical environmentalism backfires on American families, raises the prices of everyday goods and services, and discourages economic growth."[4]

Much of the overall organic backlash has been fueled by money, Big Food money in particular. Fewer than a dozen of the largest food companies in the United States control a tremendous amount of food sales and wield an enormous amount of power.[5]

Industry lobbies and corporations have created websites to extol the virtues of conventional farming and food processing, such as findourcommonground.com, created by an agricultural marketing company on behalf of the United Soybean Board and National Corn Growers Association. According to their website, they want you to "learn how to eat fearlessly."[6,7]

Some corporations hoped that the power of mom bloggers would further their efforts. Following a 2014 BlogHer conference in San

Jose, Monsanto—the highly controversial mastermind behind many of the pesticides and genetically engineered seeds that pervade farm fields around the world—invited mom bloggers to a brunch with a $150 incentive. According to several bloggers in attendance, the event attempted to offer a positive spin on the company, which spends millions to fight against GMO labeling. Not all of the attendees bought into their claims, and the blogging that followed was varied in its support.

In a testament to the greater power of the consumer, shoppers are using their dollars and their voices to create small but meaningful change. Thanks to petitions almost 400,000 strong (and possibly the fact that Kraft's 2014 profits dropped 62 percent from the previous year), the company removed artificial food dye from its macaroni and cheese.[8]

Victories for conventional food improvements have been taking on unprecedented momentum. In the past two years alone, consumer advocacy and interest in capturing the growing health-minded market has led to General Mills eliminating artificial flavors and colors from its entire line of cereals, including classics like Lucky Charms and Trix; Taco Bell and Pizza Hut phasing out artificial preservatives and dyes; Panera ditching artificial flavors and preservatives; and Subway removing "yoga mat chemical" azodicarbonamide from its bread. Even McDonald's is shifting to cage-free eggs and launching an organic burger in Germany.[9,10,11,12,13]

At the same time, parents voting with their dollars switched to brands like Annie's Homegrown natural and organic line, known for its Cheddar Bunnies and mac & cheese. But when General Mills bought Annie's in 2014, consumers like Marissa became alarmed, afraid the organic products their kids loved would be tainted by such a large corporation.

66 I am a bit concerned about the takeover of small healthy brands by larger global corporations. But I'll continue to buy Annie's and Applegate Farms because I believe they're better than the alternatives. 99

The boom in organic food has led some of the nation's biggest food companies to acquire or take stakes in smaller organic brands. White-Wave has owned Earthbound Farm since 2013 and So Delicious since 2014. Hain Celestial acquired Ella's Kitchen and Rudi's Organic Bakery in recent years, adding them to its arsenal of well-known organic brands you may have thought were still "mom-and-pop-owned." Happy Family, Van's Natural Food, and Plum Organics are all fully or majority-owned by Big Food.

Consumers and industry insiders debate whether the influence of these big companies will be detrimental to the integrity of the small brands. On one hand, it often takes the guiding hand of a large corporation to increase distribution and reduce prices, making organic more accessible to the masses. On the other hand, there may be pressure from the big guns to weaken the national organic standards and internal company values to increase profits. This leaves parents like Carissa torn on the acquisition issue.

66 *I feel like there is tremendous potential for good here. A large company recognizes the power of an organic brand, so they acquire it and increase distribution and the products become more effectively available for the masses in stores like Walmart and Target. I do get concerned, however, about reformulations. I'm also concerned about spending money on products owned by companies who donate large amounts of money to defeat GMO labeling legislation.* 99

But Robyn O'Brien says Annie's is actually a positive example of strong leadership taking an acquisition in the right direction.

66 *Now is not the time to abandon Annie's. Now is the time to make Annie's a compass inside General Mills.* 99

John Foraker, president and former CEO of Annie's, agreed to stay on at Annie's after the $820 million sale to steer the company's transition and make a true difference in the food system. Speaking at ShiftCon 2015, a health and wellness social media conference, he said he was skeptical at the start of the acquisition discussions.

❝ *But I knew for us to make true change in the world we have to make organic a much bigger part of the food system. We said, 'If you buy Annie's, there's no compromise. We have to continue to advocate for the things that got us here, and we need to really focus on supply chain.' We thought if we can get these guys to buy into what we are doing and do it at 100 times the scale, we can make the change in the world we want.* ❞

And with plans to double organic acreage, launch certified organic bunny snacks to K–12 schools, and expand its product line, Annie's is setting an example for taking organic mainstream.

Gary Hirshberg, chairman and former president and CEO of Stonyfield Farm, has also set a trailblazing example of staying true to a company's principles in the face of changing ownership. Despite selling the majority share to Groupe Danone almost 15 years ago, the 35-year-old brand has been incomparable in its ability to make organic dairy accessible. At that same ShiftCon lecture, Hirshberg said when Stonyfield was considering selling in Walmart in the early '90s, it was a radical thing to do, but he was troubled by the price gap for organic foods.

❝ *Average people don't even have a Whole Foods near them, let alone can afford it. We never set up to be elitist food. I knew the efficiencies of Walmart's transportation system and their low-margin, high-volume model meant my organic premium would be far lower than it would at another store. I felt like we needed to be there, we needed the volume to influence the supply chain. Fortunately, Walmart had no interest in controlling what we were doing. All the fears we had from this gigantic company, it was just about making sure we had supply. It's been almost 20 years, and they've had zero influence on what we do and how we do it.* ❞

Not every merger and acquisition has been such smooth sailing, but Robyn says large and small companies alike know consumers keep a watchful eye. She says the transparency and accountability social media brings to this has totally shifted power and changed the conversation.

And with that, Annie's Cheddar Bunnies are becoming the new Goldfish. It's a giant step for cheesy crackers and a small step for families across the country.

The best news is evidence that all the effort we put into instilling healthy values is not for naught. Parents like Orly who laid down ground rules for their young children have found that saying no to Oreos isn't automatically fuel for teenage rebellion.

“ *Now that my children are young adults [18 and 21], I've had the benefit of seeing how my healthy snacks policy has panned out. My oldest son recently told me that I'd spoiled him from ever enjoying the really bad snacks because he just couldn't acquire a taste.* **”**

LaToya says for her teenage daughter, the visible results of an unhealthy diet are their own coercion.

“ *She has also noticed that if she drinks a soda or eats too many sugary snacks she may get a pimple, and at 13 that consequence is greater than any FDA warning.* **”**

While organic is gradually becoming more affordable and accessible, it's simply not always an option. I've often wondered about the choice between an organic processed snack and fresh conventional produce. Should I be more concerned with ingesting pesticides or acquiring whole-food nutrition?

Jill Nussinow, registered dietitian and author of the *Veggie Queen* book series, says if it comes down to getting the food conventionally or not getting it at all, just eat the produce.

“ *If buying organic can be done, it should be, because we know that pesticides, fungicides, and herbicides aren't good for you. If you are concerned about GMOs, buying organic is also your best bet. But just getting fruits and vegetables is equally important.* **”**

The Quest for Dietary Perfection

You keep bees to produce your own honey and chickens to lay your own eggs. You never purchase anything grown more than 100 miles away.

When you're not cooking from scratch, you will only buy from small, mom-and-pop brand organic companies who have not "sold out" to large corporations. You purchase your beef from a cowshare.

You belong to a CSA and use a breadmaker. You make your own yogurt and know what a scoby is.

You try to at least buy the "dirty dozen" produce organic, but occasionally fail. You believe that if it's sold at Whole Foods, it's probably OK to eat.

You do the best you can to provide healthy meals for your family, but don't obsess over organic. You purchase processed food in bulk.

Canned ham. Hot dog-stuffed pizza. Circus peanuts. You will pretty much eat anything if it is cheap and convenient.

Leah Segedie, founder of Mamavation, a healthy living campaign for families, agrees that whole foods trump processed.

66 *I'd choose the conventional whole food, but I'd wash it a ton. I'm still of the belief that whole foods trump processed. But because 85 percent of what my kids eat is organic or non-GMO at our home, I feel more confident they will be fine with an apple from a convenience store.* 99

Considering our parents never had to think twice about a TV dinner, the maze of food is unfairly confusing for modern parents. Mom Lurena is frustrated by the general lack of oversight and clarity in labeling.

66 *It takes a ton of time and a lot of digging to get to the truth of whether a food is actually safe. It shouldn't be that way. Eggs are especially hard to figure out. Is the egg injected with antibiotics? What's the difference between free-range and organic? It's like a state secret trying to figure out what is safe or not—and forget about GMOs. You have to be persistent and determined, and it takes a ton of time and investigation to try and figure out the best and safest foods.* 99

Meanwhile, Lurena stands by her hard lines against fast food and soda. For now, she knows her three-year-old can't complain if he doesn't know what he's missing. And I have shared those same hard lines with my six-year-old son, knowing eventually he's going to be independent enough to make his own food decisions.

Carolyn says she's trying to teach her six-year-old daughter to make the right decisions, but she lets her partake in chips and cupcakes at parties and school because she doesn't want her to be "an outcast."

66 *As the school bus drove away yesterday, I saw her sneaking Fruit Loops in the backseat with her girlfriends.* 99

No matter what priorities you make for your family, being a parent means knowing that rules are meant to be broken. Personally,

I don't want my son to live his whole life without tasting a Krispy Kreme donut. But if I can get him to wash it down with some organic kale juice, I'll feel a little bit better about any transgressions.

T I P S for Buying Fruits and Veggies

☑ Not all experts or consumers agree on the priority of organic versus local. Do you buy the organic berries imported from Chile or the local conventional ones? Personally, I try to shop seasonally to avoid having to purchase organic fruit from halfway across the globe.

☑ Keep in mind that vendors at farmers' markets may be using sustainable farming methods but be unable to pay for organic certification. Always ask.

☑ The Environmental Working Group releases annual lists of the "Dirty Dozen and Clean Fifteen"—the fruits and vegetables most and least likely to contain pesticides. You can download a handy app (ewg.org/foodnews) to keep track, and you'll usually notice that apples, berries, and stone fruits like peaches tend to top the dirty list.

☑ It's also a good idea to go organic with anything where you eat the skin. Notice that avocado, kiwis, and pineapple are on the low pesticide risk list, partly because you'll be removing that inedible rind where much of the nasty stuff lives.

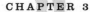

CHAPTER 3

The Precarious World of Poo Maintenance

Trickier Than Changing a Diaper With One Hand Tied Behind Your Back

MY LIFE IN DIAPERS (using, not wearing)—a brief timeline.

2009: My son is born, and the idea of cloth diapers is both foreign and repulsive.

2010: After a year of having my eco-cred criticized, I employ a local cloth diaper service and enjoy cloth diapering for the remainder of toilet training.

2013: My daughter is born with a stash of cloth diapers prepared and a washing service prepaid.

2014: The diaper service folds, and I enlist the help of my part-time nanny for laundry assistance. All continues to run smoothly.

2015: My daughter starts preschool at 18 months, eliminating the need for a nanny but leaving me with full-time laundry duty in addition to running a full-time business. On top of that, the preschool has instated a no-cloth-diaper policy. I am both annoyed and relieved. I secretly hated lugging those dirty diapers home from school. I know I can still use cloth diapers for nights and weekends but give myself permission to sell them off, hoping she will be early to potty train. (She is not.)

The disposable diaper was born in the mid-20th century. But since that time, many eco-minded parents stuck with cloth diapers to help reduce the major landfill contribution of diapers.

The Real Diaper Industry Association (RDIA), a cloth diaper advocacy group founded in 2004, estimates that 27.4 billion disposable diapers are used each year in the United States, which according to the Environmental Protection Agency translates into more than 3.4 million tons of waste dumped into landfills.

However, in the past 20 years, several studies on cloth vs. disposable have sparked debate over whether opting for cloth has any real environmental impact.

While one study in the early '90s touted the environmental superiority of reusable diapers, another found no significant difference in impact when considering the water and energy used to launder cloth diapers. Both studies have faced criticism, in no small part because each was sponsored by an invested group—The National Association of Diaper Services, a trade association affiliated with RDIA, and Procter & Gamble, the maker of Pampers.[1,2]

A 2008 study by the UK Environment Agency and Department for Environment, Food and Rural Affairs confused matters a bit more, stating reusable diapers can cause significantly less or significantly more damage to the environment than disposable ones, depending on how parents wash and dry them.[3]

I've seen what the average child can produce. Unless you are outside with a washboard, a clothesline, and plenty of time, it would be hard not to use a substantial amount of water and energy to clean cloth diapers. After using cloth diapers for the first six months of her child's life, water was mom Marissa's main concern.

&& *The problem was not only the time spent but the amount of water and energy I used with the pre-wash and then wash cycle every two to three days. I really felt like I'd be doing the planet a favor by switching to disposable (and it gave me an extra half hour every other day) when he started eating solid foods and the messes were even harder to clean out.* 99

Disposable may make life easier for parents tasked with washing and drying, but there are still no studies that truly factor water and energy versus the entire life cycle of a conventional disposable diaper.

Dr. Alan Greene, author of *Raising Baby Green*, a handbook for holistic moms, writes that though the Environment Agency report is more thorough than other analyses to date, it is still quite incomplete. He cites the study's omission of greener alternative diaper brands, as well as its failure to examine the entire lifeline of the manufacturing process—the oil rigs that yield plastic liners, the forests where the wood pulp starts as trees, and the cotton fields where the cloth is born. Greene concludes that any diaper choice will have an unavoidable impact on the environment, but we can make choices to lessen the burden.

Ways to lower the environmental impact of cloth diapers include using an eco-friendly detergent, choosing renewable resources like cotton and wool over synthetic fibers, and reusing them for another child. Fortunately, some great advances have been made for more eco-friendly disposables. "Hybrid diapers" like gDiapers and Kushies make flushable liners for reusable outer diapers. And brands like Seventh Generation, Nature Babycare, and Earth's Best manufacture chlorine-free diapers made with somewhat more sustainable resources than conventional diapers. They are not a cure-all, but are certainly a compromise for people who want to minimize the burden on landfills without having to wash cloth diapers.

It was such a compromise with Dad that made actress Alysia Reiner call it quits with the cloth. Who knew husbands were so squeamish?

❝ *We ended up with chlorine-free disposables. My husband is a very neat, clean man, and it just didn't work for him and it wasn't worth it for me.* **❞**

New mom Abby says her husband was pleasantly surprised after being worried about using cloth.

❝ My husband was really worried about the prospect of having to wash poopy diapers in our washing machine. But he became a huge believer once he saw how easy and cost-effective it was. I have now walked in on him having numerous conversations with his dad friends trying to sell them on trying it out. ❞

Not deterred by any naysayers, mom Stephanie was determined to not only use cloth diapers but also be sure everything that touched her daughter's skin would be free of chemicals from the second she was born. For baby's first bath at the hospital, she provided the organic soap, organic towels, organic clothing, and cloth diapers.

❝ People would say: 'I just can't imagine doing that. It must be sooo hard.' It actually pisses me off a bit because it is not that much extra work. We rarely have leaks or diaper rash, and I'm doing my part to help my daughter's future by reducing waste. ❞

Still, for parents like Meghan, it's not so much the idea of extra work but the idea of tainting their washing machines.

❝ I use disposable diapers for both of my children. If my kids have a blowout, the outfit goes in the garbage. I just cannot fathom putting poop in my washer, the same one that washes dishcloths and towels and washcloths. I almost convinced my husband to buy me a second washer just for cloth diapers, because it does intrigue me, but I just can't get over myself. ❞

The simplest cloth diaper solution for the squeamish is the local diaper service, which handles all the dirty work for you. They drop off a stash of perfectly fitted diapers right to your door. They also take the whole mess away, carrying your dirty diapers back to their place to clean and sanitize. And the best part is that even with this door-to-door service, you can still save up to $1,500 on the average diaperhood. You can find a diaper service near you at diaperservice .realdiaperindustry.org.

Doing a dirty diaper wash on your own isn't terribly difficult either, especially if you use all-in-ones. Since you knock off most of the solid mess into the toilet, just do a rinse cycle and then a regular cycle with a good green detergent. (Some people do an extra rinse at the end.) The diapers often come out spotless.

But mom Monica found that some daycares and preschools give parents a hard time about using cloth at their facilities, often simply out of unfamiliarity.

" *I asked if our daycare was cloth-diaper-friendly, and they were not. I understood from doing research that apparently in Pennsylvania, one supposedly has the right to ask the daycare to use any kind of diaper the parent provides. However, I didn't want to get into an argument with the otherwise ideal daycare or annoy the daycare providers by making them do something 'different,' so I just sucked it up and we switched to disposables.* **"**

Fortunately, Jeanette didn't face that same obstacle with the daycare she chose in that same state.

" *My daycare was totally open to cloth diapers. It was a bit of a learning curve to explain the assembly, but was thereafter very straightforward. They even went above and beyond the call of duty and rinsed and separated out the soiled ones for us every day.* **"**

For the ultimate in eco-friendly parenting, there exists an option that entirely forgoes the need for any landfill waste in the diaper department: elimination communication. A common practice of the "attachment parenting" movement, this trending technique uses timing, signals, and cues to potty train infants from birth. Advocates like Mayim Bialik—the über-crunchy mom formerly known as Blossom—tout the benefits of avoiding conventional diapering. Yet for moms like Bonnie, it sounds hard to believe.

" *Is elimination communication for real? I've read about it, but no friends or neighbors have ever brought it up in conversation. It sounds like an urban legend, like people who supposedly potty train their cats.* **"**

I also thought it sounded completely insane—until I met down-to-earth mom and personal trainer Jessi.

Jessi's first experience with early potty training came at a babysitting gig when the mother informed her that her ten-month-old son would prefer to poop on the potty. Shocked by the child's young age, pregnant Jessi looked online to find out just how early one could really begin toilet training. She discovered the diaper-free movement, ordered a DVD, and sat in on a local meeting where she was pleased to see another mom with a Prada handbag.

66 *There were all kinds of moms, from major hippies to women wearing couture. One lady from Eastern Europe said her family back home was appalled that her first child was still in diapers at age one. The US is the only country so dependent on diapers.* **99**

It's true that most babies in other countries are trained well before their second birthday. In fact, in the first half of the 20th century, before the advent of disposable diapers, most American children were toilet trained by 18 months.

Jessi cites the waste-free, green aspect of elimination communication as one of its draws, as well as a smoother transition to official potty training.

66 *I see this sort of as a potty-training prequel. I don't catch every single pee or poo, and I use gDiapers for insurance. I'm taking a part-time approach, especially with the transition to a daycare where the workers may not be as supportive of taking Gigi to the potty. My family was skeptical at first, but they have embraced it and rush to put her on the potty.* **99**

While Jessi's experience was favorable, with her daughter taking to the cues and signals at four days old, elimination communication doesn't work for everyone. Chrissy tried her hand at it when her daughter was nine months old and found the result to be less than environmentally friendly.

  66 *I figured if I could teach her to use the potty, then I would be doing the greenest thing of all. My child wouldn't need diapers anymore, and my constant attention to her bathroom body language was bound to create a bond between us. Well, Mama didn't pay as much attention as I should have, and my daughter ended up going to the bathroom, only not just on the potty. Don't get me wrong, she used the potty several times successfully. However, she also used the family room rugs and the kitchen floor more times than the she did the potty. After countless tiffs with the hubby, I decided to let this one go and just stuck with the cloth diapers. I actually think I ended up wasting more of our precious earth's resources because I needed to have the rugs cleaned twice during a few months.* 99

True—if you're spending more resources cleaning up from accidents than cleaning up the diapers, elimination communication may not be for you. In the diaper debate, we have no clear answers. Most environmentalists agree that it comes down to what's best for Mom and Dad, and getting a divorce over dirty nappies isn't going to help anybody.

T I P S for Diaper Duty

☑ You can locate a local cloth diaper service at diaperservice
.realdiaperindustry.org/locate-a-diaper-service. There are
also dozens of online resources with tips on cleaning your
own cloth diapers.

☑ If your daycare center or preschool isn't on board with the
cloth diapering, the Real Diaper Association offers tips for
introducing cloth diapers to a daycare center: realdiaper
association.org/daycare/daycare-tip-sheet.pdf.

☑ If you choose to use disposables, there are now dozens of
fragrance- and chlorine-free brands on the market using
more sustainable resources, including Honest, Seventh
Generation, Nature Babycare, and Earth's Best.

☑ If you are interested in elimination communication,
diaperfreebaby.org offers a network of free support groups.

CHAPTER 4

Your Breast Friend— Or Worst Enemy?

Making the Most of What Nature Gave You

SOMEWHERE BETWEEN the formula revolution of the 1970s and the modern green movement, there came a heavily renewed interest in the benefits of breastfeeding. Shortly after the moment of conception, total strangers will ask you if you plan to nurse.

It's a noble ambition and certainly among the "greenest" things a mother can do. After all, it relieves the need for massive cans of formula and hundreds of dishwasher runs for bottles.

With all my best intentions, I was fairly certain breastfeeding would not come easy for me. Just about everyone I knew had difficulties, from sore, cracked nipples to an actual fatal case of infection from mastitis.

I took a breastfeeding class while I was pregnant that drilled into parents the horrors of "nipple confusion." I was told that if I wanted this to work I had to be ready for 24/7 feeding—there would be no rest for the weary.

That first night in the hospital after giving birth a nurse offered to feed my son a bottle of formula so I could get a solid three or four hours of sleep. I was appalled by her offer—hadn't she ever heard of nipple confusion?

Reassured and exhausted, I relented and let her give my baby a bottle. Blessedly, when returned to breast, my son didn't miss a beat.

They say breast size is irrelevant, but I believe that I was given those double Ds (*past tense*) for a reason. Coupled with my abnormally high prolactin levels, my milk flowed like the river Jordan. This, it seemed, was an endeavor in which I was quite skilled.

In fact, I was so enthralled with my gift for lactation, I dreamed about joining with Salma Hayek to nurse starving children in Africa. Determined to make good on some mitzvah karma, I posted on a few forums where people search for breast milk donations for adopted children. I offered up my freezer stash for people coming cross-country to pick up their newborns, several of whom had been born to drug-addicted parents.

But, after a full disclosure of my medications, even the parents of heroin-weaned babies didn't want my Zoloft-laced milk.

Yes, I took Zoloft, an anti-anxiety medication, through my pregnancy and seven months of nursing. The general medical consensus seemed to be that a few selective serotonin reuptake inhibitors in breast milk still outweigh formula.

Issues with nursing—either with the act itself or anxiety about what said milk may contain—are one of the most common guilt-inducing, panic-striking subjects for new mothers. A Google search for "breastfeeding problems" yields 30.5 million results. And if that's not enough to keep you busy with worry, try "breastfeeding and medication" for well over 32 million hits.

The pressure to breastfeed begins well before the baby looks for its first meal. Modern mothers like actress Alysia Reiner attended breastfeeding classes and workshops while pregnant, trying to get a jumpstart on lactation and latching.

❝ *My parents thought it was weird that I went to a class, watched a video, had a doula give me tips, and had the phone number of five lactation consultants. They're saying, 'It's the most natural thing in the world, what's your problem?' Meanwhile, neither of them did it.* ❞

Teeming with pre-childbirth nursing anxiety, Amy Wilson, actress and author of *When Did I Get Like This?*, feels like she only fueled her apprehension by attending a breastfeeding support group.

> ❝ *I left that meeting horrified at the stories of mastitis and thrush, certain that I would never succeed—but also more certain than ever that I had no choice but to try, since the alternative (formula) was unthinkable. As it turned out, I had a really positive breastfeeding experience, after a typically rocky first week or two. But it was hampered by the notion that any bottle, even one bottle of pumped breast milk, could threaten everything I had worked so hard to create. I think we do new mothers a real disservice by telling them it has to be all-or-nothing with breastfeeding.* ❞

After the classes, books, videos, and hundreds of dollars spent on pumps and hands-free nursing bras, the true test begins as mothers battle thrush, mastitis, cracked nipples, tied tongues, colic, milk allergies, and sheer exhaustion from being a 24-hour milk machine.

Comedian Tammy Pescatelli says when she came home from the hospital after having her son, she was depressed because she had trouble with nursing and was struggling with her decision.

> ❝ *I was so emotional and hysterical that I went online to one of those forums. I was talking about the guilt of not breastfeeding and how I wanted to. Within hours, the La Leche League called my house and wanted to send a wet nurse over to breastfeed my baby. I said, 'My baby's fine, but my husband could use some attention.'* ❞

With raw nipples and minimal milk production, Corina called breastfeeding the worst experience of her life.

> ❝ *Every time I went to hold my son, the poor thing went rooting for my breast. He was probably starving, but I couldn't breastfeed as much as he wanted because I was in so much pain. It kept me from holding my baby and actually caused me to resent him a little bit. After six weeks, I finally started with formula and actually got some sleep and the baby had a full belly. I still feel guilty about not sticking with it longer because there's so much pressure out there. But if I had to do it again, I would try to be the best mom for my family instead of trying to be a hero. If that means switching to formula instead of breastfeeding, then that's OK.* ❞

Dr. Mark Diamond, a Pittsburgh-based pediatrician who regularly teaches a baby basics class to new and expecting parents, says that while there are clear physical benefits of breastfeeding, it needs to be emotionally satisfying for the mother.

66 *If you don't want to breastfeed because it's painful or physically or emotionally taxing, but you feel obligated, the baby picks up on that and feels your tension and body language. If a mother is upset, babies can sense that and it puts stress on the baby. Do the benefits of nursing outweigh the stress induced by these other factors? Professionally, I don't think they do.* 99

Diamond says he certainly encourages moms to nurse and believes it is the best way to go, but he says we are fortunate to have a reasonable alternative with formula. Most doctors would agree there's no right answer for every scenario.

Mothers like Jennifer who need to go back to the office after a mere six weeks of maternity leave have the added aggravation of pumping milk throughout the day while another caregiver gets to do the feeding.

66 *My baby latched right away. The struggle I experienced was when I went back to work. There is never a convenient time to pump, and the reward is so intangible, as a teacher at daycare gives her the bottles every day so I'm missing all of that bonding time. But I keep reminding myself that it's what is best for my daughter, so at ten months I'm still pumping.* 99

Where it used to be a matter of modesty to publicly nurse, the current judgment from other mothers is enough for mom Rebecca to feel ashamed any time her baby *wasn't* latched to her breast.

66 *I used to feel conspicuous when feeding my first baby pumped breast milk in public in case anyone thought I was giving her formula.* 99

Sarah had no problem nursing her first child. But due to her second child's temperament, she has no qualms about formula supplementation.

❝ *He's sensitive to dairy, so I cut dairy out of my diet. If he's worked up, overtired, or his sister is in the room, he won't latch. He only nurses for maybe five minutes per side. If he's fussing and I turn to nursing, he doesn't take comfort in it. He gets one or two soy formula bottles a day now during those worked-up fits or overtired moments when he won't latch. I don't have any guilt about formula. I definitely want to nurse him, and I don't intend to quit. He's just not making it easy on me. The soy bottles take a little pressure off my shoulders. I'm relieved I have something to turn to when he won't latch.* ❞

When the obstacles are surmountable, we soldier on, proud of ourselves for succeeding in a task that isn't so easy after all. We know the indisputable benefits of nutrition, immunities—and my personal favorite—weight loss. But after nine months of diligently watching everything we put in or on our bodies (and freaking out after accidentally huffing nitrous oxide while trying to suck the remaining whipped cream out of the can), we face months or years of similar conscientiousness as a sole source of nourishment.

When I had my second baby, I resolved to nurse for closer to a year. And it was a good thing I had favorable plans in place, because three years later things had changed at the hospital.

The hospital installed a new "baby-friendly" policy to encourage breastfeeding. It was wonderful that nurses made the effort to educate new parents and promote lactation by encouraging "rooming in" with baby. But I was struck by the drastic change in attitude toward formula supplementation. This time, when I asked a nurse to give a bottle so I could get a bit of rest, she refused. She said my husband could give a bottle, but they would not take the baby out of our room.

The first few nights were extremely difficult. Stunned awake listening for crying and trying not to take too many painkillers to ease the stitches, I felt terrified at the prospect of having another tiny human being to care for, and at the same time, completely in awe of her beauty.

Due to anxiety with a generous helping of obsessive-compulsive disorder, I remained on a low dose of Zoloft through both pregnancies. But this time it wasn't enough to get me through the hormone drop and inexplicable postpartum terror. I experienced sheer panic that I could not pin to any particular fear or reason. I was, once again, completely sure I would never sleep again.

When I got home, things got infinitely worse. Even when I had ample opportunity to sleep while my husband took the baby downstairs, I lay awake shaking with anxiety. I kept telling myself I would never get enough sleep, not be able to function, and ultimately, not be able to care for my children. It was the absolute fear of losing control coupled with the fear of having to exclusively formula feed.

I sat on the phone daily with my psychiatrist trying to find the quickest solution to get myself together. Xanax wasn't working. Even Ambien did nothing for me. The next step would be to try some medications that would make breastfeeding very risky, and I knew I'd be even more depressed if I lost the ability to nurse. (Note: both Ambien and Xanax prescription information caution against use while breastfeeding, but I discussed the risks and benefits with my doctors and did not nurse during the time when the concentration was highest.)

But I knew I had to be a functional mother first and foremost, so I began taking a small dose of Klonopin, another anti-anxiety medication with a nursing warning. I also gradually upped my Zoloft to my usual level. I was terrified that nothing would work, but that night, I finally slept soundly while my husband took care of the baby. By the next day, I was starting to feel a bit better. I also began to do more research on nursing and medications by going to the premier expert in the field, the Infant Risk Center. The counselors there agreed it should be relatively safe to temporarily take the medications at bedtime and then not nurse for a few hours while the concentrations were highest. I just had to keep a careful eye out for sedation, which fortunately I didn't experience.

I was so happy to nurse again, even if it was just part-time. Gradually, things continued to improve. After a couple days my husband

and the baby started sleeping upstairs again so we could take proper feeding shifts. I lowered my dose of Klonopin and arranged a feeding schedule where formula would fill in when my body was spiked with medication.

It was one of the hardest things I ever went through, but I know I was not alone. On top of postpartum depression, passing medicine in utero and through breast milk is a continual source of added anxiety for mothers.

Jeanette, a mother of a two-year-old, says she struggled with getting back on her "happy medication," but she was relieved when she finally made the decision to take it again.

66 *I ended up going back on medication after about four months of breastfeeding, and I'm very glad I did. I went off during pregnancy, but my doctor and I decided it was best to go back on when the need arose for me personally, which was when I was still breastfeeding. It was a tough decision weighing the pros and cons, but I decided that taking care of myself was the best way I could take care of the baby and the family. I'm so happy with the decision and will definitely stick with that decision if there is a next time as well.* 99

Due to lack of studies, inconclusiveness, or general fear of malpractice, just about everything has a warning label regarding pregnancy and nursing. And it's hard to get straight answers, even from doctors. Like me, new mom Amy got the runaround when she tried to find out if her medications were "safe."

66 *While I was nursing, I got bronchitis and freaked out about having to take an antibiotic. The doctor assured me the antibiotic and the inhaler he prescribed were compatible with nursing. When I filled the prescription for the inhaler, it said in big bold letters not to use while nursing. So I panicked and didn't use it. It's so hard to get accurate information about what's safe during breastfeeding. I'm not sure if it's because doctors are too busy or don't want to be accountable. Before the bronchitis was diagnosed, I was trying to figure out what over-the-counter cold medicine was safe to take. I called my OB. They said to call the pediatrician.*

I called the pediatrician. They said to call the OB. So I gave up, and that's probably part of the reason I got bronchitis. **"**

Amy says if the American Academy of Pediatrics is going to push breastfeeding, pediatricians need to be better trained on mother's health issues during nursing. And if the pediatricians won't do it, the obstetricians should. Like many mothers, she is fed up with having to rely on the contradictory internet for medical information.

Sharon, a mother and nurse, echoes the frustration that many prescribers are not up to date on the latest studies on breastfeeding and medication.

" *Pump and dump is not necessary as often as many doctors say. I hope that more providers are checking the latest evidence-based research.* **"**

Dr. Diamond says the root of the problem is that often there really is no answer—many things have never been studied, so the honest answer is that doctors don't know.

" *When a parent asks if she can take something, the first question is, has anyone studied the effect of maternal ingestion on the baby, and in a lot of situations, the answer is no. There are a lot of generalizations and extrapolations but without any data. So a lot of times the doctor really doesn't know, and the safest answer is to say, 'If possible, don't take it.'* **"**

However, researchers have studied a number of the drugs out there, Diamond says. It's just that some doctors don't know what information is available.

" *As a physician, my answer is that if I don't know the answer I'll find it. Some doctors don't want to take the time to do that so they pass it along to the next guy. Everybody passes the buck a little bit. But for many drugs, there is just no knowledge. You can only go by the information you have at hand.* **"**

According to the website of the illustrious Dr. Bill Sears—father of eight children, as well as the author of more than 30 books on childcare—what physicians tell moms about taking a medication while breastfeeding is based more on legal considerations than scientific knowledge.[1]

❝ *The information available from pharmaceutical companies about a drug often advises mothers not to breastfeed while taking a drug, but this advice reflects the company's desire to protect itself from lawsuits and to avoid having to do expensive research that would allow it to say a certain drug is safe.* ❞

Sears says healthcare providers advising nursing mothers should rely on additional sources of information, like the extensive online Infant Risk Breastfeeding and Medications Forum administered by Dr. Thomas Hale, professor of pediatrics at Texas Tech University.[2]

As for the occasional over-the-counter remedy, the general consensus of the medical community seems to be that "breast is best," as long as you avoid the hard stuff (i.e., streamlining cocaine, doing multiple tequila shots, or pounding raw eggs). Though she worries about the toxins in her home, mom Rebecca felt confident in her body's chemistry and didn't feel highly encumbered by the limitations of nursing her children over a year.

❝ *I never had a moment's hesitation about what my breast milk contained. I figured that unless I was using drugs, drinking, or actually eating BPA plastic containers, breast milk was the best choice, hands down.* ❞

But not all moms are so confident in the ability of their own bodies to produce the healthiest beverage. As far back as 1951, scientists reported finding pesticides in breast milk. PBDE flame-retardants and mercury are also among the contaminants often found in breast milk, which essentially tells the story of the mother's life exposure to chemicals.[3]

But Dr. Diamond says that while breast milk does carry environmental contaminants and we don't know what all their effects are, breastfeeding is still the superior choice.

❝ *For all the benefits of breastfeeding, nobody has been able to demon-strate that the trace amounts of these things make that much of a differ-ence. There's nothing showing up in the breast milk at this point that has been proven in any way to seriously hurt the baby. Even organic formula can't begin to match the benefits of the immunity and brain-developing components of breast milk.* **❞**

Knowing these benefits, whether we stop after one fitful night in the hospital or well into toddlerhood, it can be hard to let go.

After eight months of nursing, pumping, occasionally supple-menting, and constantly *brexting* (a new thing to feel guilty about—using a smartphone during feeding, which some experts have cautioned may affect mother-child bonding), I made the difficult decision to stop nursing. Years later, I worry I stopped for terribly selfish reasons—a desire to wear a bathing suit without nursing pads, not bringing a pump on vacation, the misguided idea that it would help me lose the last few pounds of baby weight. Mostly, it was to let go of the remaining anxiety. I was still terrified by the pills I had to take to keep myself sane, constantly questioning Tylenol for a headache and sunny-side-up eggs for fear of salmonella.

I truly did enjoy breastfeeding. Maybe even more this time around. In addition to all the health benefits I knew my daughter re-ceived, I felt that close connection and enjoyed the ease of not having to make bottles or spend money on formula. I even found it *relaxing*.

But the relaxation was fleeting, and more often, the concern over the long-term effect of my actions plagued me. I was damned if I did and damned if I didn't. And since I stopped, I've felt a pang of sadness anytime I see a baby at a woman's breast. But mom Liz says I'm certainly not the only one.

❝ *I don't know any Jewish mother who doesn't inherently suffer from guilt. I feel like if I breastfed until my kid was in college I would still feel guilty that I stopped too soon and that I was a terrible mom.* **❞**

If you can't give kudos to yourself for being a perfectly organic milk machine, try to remember the new generation of mothers has something going for it that is true "liquid gold"—awareness. We may not know everything, but at least we know *better* than we did ten years ago. So if we can't be perfect mamas, at least we can be smart ones.

T I P S for Breast and Bottle Feeding

☑ The Infant Risk Hotline (infantrisk.com) is the most extensive resource for evidence-based research on breastfeeding and medication, and their free hotline offers helpful and non-judgmental information. Their new website mommymeds.com is based upon the same rigorous research, studies, and experience of the InfantRisk Center, presented in a user-friendlier manner.

☑ If you do use formula, look for organic brands. Not all organic brands are created equal, but at least you know their milk does not come from cows that were fed GMO feed, given antibiotics, or injected with synthetic growth hormones. Additionally, organic formula's sweeteners and oils cannot be GMO, treated with pesticides, or extracted with neurotoxic solvents.

☑ Did you know you are probably entitled to a free breast pump through the Affordable Health Care Act (aka Obamacare)? Neither did most of the moms I talked to. This program started in August 2010, shortly before I became pregnant with my second child, and it took a lot of calling and insisting to insurance company representatives before I finally obtained one. Some moms said it couldn't have been easier for them to have a free quality pump shipped to their doorstep, while some gave up after getting the runaround. Fortunately, now there are websites to ease the process, like medelabreastfeedingus.com /insurance-pump-lookup.

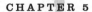

CHAPTER 5

How About I Just Let Them Go Naked?

**Shopping for Itty-Bitty Socks
Used to Be Much More Fun**

AT THE CRUX of the environmental crisis is a planet consumed with consumption. We just love stuff—especially new, shiny stuff to replace the old, out-of-style, worn-out stuff. But the dangerous result of our addiction to this vicious cycle is clearly displayed in Annie Leonard's viral internet film *The Story of Stuff*.

Leonard's film examines the real costs of our consumer-driven culture, including the consumption of resources and subsequent waste elimination. She also observes society's obsession with consumption, stemming from changing trends and a bit of innate greed. Critics have panned the video as anti-capitalist and anti-consumer— even anti-American. But its core thesis—"you cannot run a linear system on a finite planet indefinitely"—has inspired screenings from elementary schools to corporate sustainability training across the globe.

Despite our growing awareness of the evils of consumption, we can't help the simple fact that kids need stuff. Their clothing size changes faster than your mind about squeezing into those "jeggings." And unless you have a generous supply of hand-me-downs, you are going to have to somehow procure basic necessities for your child.

Where ten years back we may have been quick to throw away worn-out shoes or a torn T-shirt, many mothers are reverting to the sewing and mending ways of our grandmothers. If we can't find a way to fix it, we find a way to reuse, repurpose, or recycle—anything to keep merchandise out of the landfills.

While hand-me-downs might have been a shameful secret for kids and parents alike back in the excess heydays of the '80s and '90s, it's become quite acceptable, and even hip, to shop the secondhand stores. And that's good news for the environment, as research on the hierarchy on sustainability shows secondhand reigns supreme.

I am a pro at scoring free secondhand clothing for my children. In fact, I consider my clothing savings a way to make up for the extra money I spend on organic food.

Moms like Rebecca prefer used clothes because, in addition to being cost-effective and resourceful, they've been washed many times, removing a good amount of the chemical finishings and dyes.

❝ I refuse to buy clothing that's been treated with flame retardants or stain/wrinkle-resistant treatments. I will buy those at consignment shops and wash them in natural detergent with a cup of vinegar added just to be on the safer side. ❞

Actress Alysia Reiner also favors hand-me-downs and enjoys the "circle of motherhood," giving and receiving items.

❝ If it's not organic, at least they've washed it a bunch of times so a lot of the yucky stuff is gone. ❞

Sandra, a mother of two, agrees—the more hand-me-downs the better.

❝ We are blessed to have several families giving clothing to my daughter. She burns right through them, and I pass them along to other families for continued use. It's a great budget-saving strategy, and I feel good about the reuse. ❞

And if you don't have bags of clothes magically appearing at your door, mom Honi says it never hurts to ask around.

❝ *When we need something specific, I just ask friends on Facebook. I just got four pairs of cleats from one Facebook post.* ❞

Latoya, mom of a 13-year-old, says she has actually found that sometimes the giver is more thankful than the recipient.

❝ *Sometimes it's about making the person feel good that they have something to give.* ❞

For us, super cute and easy play clothes came and went without a hitch until the start of kindergarten—and the dreaded uniform. Yes, even at my city's public school, a basic uniform is required. In my son's case, he must wear navy pants and a white collared shirt, which I consider to be extremely poor choices for two reasons. Navy pants are not as easy to come by secondhand, and white shirts just scream to be regularly destroyed and replaced.

I really didn't want to buy these new clothes and searched for hand-me-downs all around, but most of the parents I knew were in the khaki-pants school zone. I waited until the last minute, hoping for a white shirt windfall. Until, alas, I had to suck it up and hit the back-to-school sale at Old Navy. I bought four pants, three shorts, and eight shirts for under $100. It was cheap—almost *too* cheap.

The force behind these low prices is the "fast fashion" model, popularized by retail giants such as H&M, Zara, and Forever 21. Fast fashion is dependent on shifting trends at a rapid pace and has become associated with disposable fashion because it delivers of-the-moment style to the mass market at a low price.

Amy DuFault, sustainable fashion writer and consultant, says fast fashion's problem is that by speeding up the rate of everything from production to trends, we are seeing massively altered systems that are breaking down.

❝ *Garment workers are putting in more time than ever led by bosses competing with the production house next door that is offering ten cents less. Subcontracting, the Wild West of apparel production, is so normal that it can't be regulated. So, in addition to unsafe and unethical working conditions for adults, child labor, which consists of more than 200 million children, is thriving.* **99**

Fast fashion also creates an abundance of textile waste. According to the EPA, the United States alone generates 14.3 million tons of used textile waste per year. In addition to having to deal with the challenge of where to put the discarded clothing, we need to take a closer look at the natural resources involved in the creation of all this clothing.

According to the Danish Fashion Institute (2013), fashion is the world's second most polluting industry, only bested by oil.[1]

And Amy sees no chance of fast fashion slowing down.

66 *As long as consumers demand it and think they deserve cheap, fast fashion, the industry will thrive like fast food. It's an exceptional business model—except for the fact that we have some serious environmental issues that will eventually force fast fashion to pull the reins back.* **99**

Large brands like H&M have made some efforts to improve sustainability, though a 2013 factory fire in Bangladesh left its manufacturing practices in question. Walmart has an affordable organic line of baby clothing, but it is made in China. There are hundreds of smaller niche organic and made-in-the-USA brands for children's clothing—though they just might charge you $75 for a onesie.

Amy says we should be considering both quality and the expected wear and lifespan of an item.

66 *Think about the usage of that garment. Will you wear it a lot? If you were to break it down to cost per wear, would it seem like you got your money's worth?* **99**

When it comes to buying new, Sandra understands the labor and environmental issues for fair trade and organic. But she says she just can't justify paying the hefty prices for children's clothes.

❝ *For my own clothes, I'm willing to invest in fair-trade items and organic cotton T-shirts because I will use them for a long time. For the kids, I can't convince myself to make this choice since they lose, soil, and outgrow clothing so quickly. I hate to admit it, but I do buy my kids' clothes from mainstream retailers. It's not a choice I'm proud of, but I haven't hit the tipping point yet that will drive my purchase in a new eco-direction.* ❞

Elizabeth agrees that she would love to buy locally made, organic clothes exclusively but can't find many reasonably priced options.

❝ *Let's face it, kids grow fast, so the budget is king. The only approach that makes sense is to buy from a consignment shop. If organic children's clothes were made at a reasonable price, I would make the switch and buy them. Then I could send them to the consignment shop when she has outgrown them.* ❞

But lack of money or quality consignment—and sometimes just resignation to accepting receipt-less gifts—often leaves parents with more conventionally made baby clothes than they'd prefer. Every time we dress our kids up in those adorable matching jumpers adorned with friendly cartoon characters, we wince at the thought of the underage factory worker's hands that knit the seams.

We know that organic is better because of the sustainable farming practices. We know that "Made in the USA" is better because less travel reduces the item's carbon footprint. But finding clothes—let alone children's clothes—that adhere to both those standards is like finding a needle in a pesticide-ridden haystack. And finding ones in a reasonable price range is sadly that much harder.

Organic cotton baby clothes have hefty prices for three reasons. First, natural pest removal and fertilizer methods simply cost more. Second, the quality of organic cotton clothing is higher. Not exposed to harsh chemicals during the growing and harvesting process, organic cotton fibers are thicker, softer, and more durable. Durability and softness can actually save money in the long run, especially when you're talking about well-worn items like sheets and blankets. But it can be tough to convince someone to spend that extra cash on clothing that a baby may only wear once.

The third reason may be the one we have most control over changing: the level of demand. Without going too deep into Economics 101, higher demand = larger supply = lower cost.

Stephanie says she tried to find clothes that met all the criteria of the conscious mother: organic, locally made, and fair trade. Unfortunately, the pickings were slim, and she could barely find even conventional clothes that weren't manufactured overseas.

66 *I am often torn with buying organic clothes made in foreign countries or buying non-organic made-in-the-USA clothes. Some big box stores and fast fashion chains now sell organic lines of baby clothing, but they are made overseas. However, it is really affordable and doesn't cost any more than regular baby clothes. So, I hate to say it, but I did buy some of these clothes because they were organic. I feel really guilty at the same time because I know they have a much larger carbon footprint than made in the USA. And who knows if there are children in sweatshops making these clothes?* 99

But when it comes to new non-organic clothing, she makes no apologies about taking them back.

66 *If someone buys me new non-organic clothes, I will sell them to a consigner or return them to the store if I have a receipt. I have no shame in that respect.* 99

Jill Ouellette, chair and professor of the fashion marketing program at Northwood University in Midland, MI, says Stephanie is right to value organic materials over local production. She says when faced with the choice between the apparel material sources or the origin of manufacture, organic is the best choice.

66 *Conventional cotton is the most polluting agricultural crop in the world. Chemicals used on conventional cottons are not only horribly*

harmful to the environment, they contain carcinogens. Although there are handling rules in the US, India, for example, allows for unrestricted use of chemicals. Therefore, not only is the environment being harmed, farmers can get cancer and suffer due to the lack of regulation on the chemicals used. **99**

Because organic cotton is more costly to produce, companies keep costs down by producing overseas. Ouellette says that if consumers in the United States hold out for wider availability of products that are both organic and locally made, they will unfortunately be waiting a long time.

66 *If the US decreases its desire for consumer products at a low cost, then perhaps manufacturing will come back to the US. But until then, focus on buying organic.* **99**

She also cites the excellent apparel performance properties and sustainability of hemp and bamboo. But she warns that while these materials are generally organic when grown, not all bamboo and hemp is treated sustainably in the production process. Even organic cotton can be treated with harmful dyes, but Ouellette says the No. 1 material and label to look for is still organic cotton.

If you can only afford to buy one organic clothing item for your children, go with pajamas—after all, those are the items they are spending 10 to 15 hours per day in. Zulily.com is a great place to find big sales on organic pajamas. I recently bought my son two pairs of deeply discounted organic Christmas pajamas despite the fact we are actually Jewish.

As with all purchases, we place our votes and use our voices when we spend money on clothing. Ideally, we'd be taking a strong stand for sustainable fibers and social justice with every exchange, but far more likely, we'll accept a mix of used bargain-bin jumpers somewhere along the way.

T I P S for Secondhand Scores

☑ I may not have nieces and nephews to hand me down their treasures, but I have become an expert at finding second-hand clothing without spending a dime.

☑ Have an older boy and younger girl? Find a family with just the opposite and arrange to swap clothing seasonally. We have friends with an older girl and younger boy, and leave bags of outgrown clothing for each other in the school cubbies. Don't know a family that fits the bill? Post your request on a local moms' board.

☑ Don't be afraid to ask. If your child has a playmate with no plans for a younger sibling, hit up the mom to see what she's doing with outgrown clothes. If she just planned on giving them to Goodwill, maybe they can go through you first.

☑ Yerdle.com and local Buy Nothing Groups are a treasure trove for free used children's clothing (and grown-up clothes too).

☑ Passed down something with a strong fabric detergent scent? Soak the clothing with one cup of white vinegar and cold water before a wash.

☑ If you can't get them free, get them cheap.

☑ Various organizations hold pop-up consignment sales or even "clothing swaps" throughout the year.

☑ Don't miss neighborhood yard sales, especially multi-family ones.

☑ Craigslist and eBay remain a mecca of trash-to-treasure bargain finds, including plenty of gently used and organic baby clothes. And new e-commerce shops and apps like Poshmark and Thredup offer deeply discounted second-hand fashion for women and children.

☑ Michelle, mom of a 13-year-old, says she learned some tips from working in a secondhand store. "Check out church rummage sales (parishioners always donate tons of kids' clothes) and school rummage sales (where there are kids, there are kids' clothes). Also, when I bring things into a consignment shop, I always take the store credit for my sales instead of cash because you usually get a substantially larger percentage. When I use it to purchase items at the store, it's like getting free clothes."

CHAPTER 6

Maybe It's Safer to Go Play in Traffic

When Knives Seem Safer Than Rubber Duckies

MY GRANDMOTHER'S favorite story about my childhood underlines the simplicity of entertaining a toddler. Apparently, I spent a long afternoon taking an empty astringent bottle in and out of a wastebasket. When my mother came to pick me up, I became inconsolable when torn away from the trash can.

While a baby probably would be content to play with a few wooden spoons and homemade sock puppets, the conventional consumer world would not tend to agree.

Eco-savvy moms may register for toys made by companies with the highest records of safety and sustainability, but a run-of-the-mill plastic toy is bound to make it into the playpen.

Every day we hear about massive recalls of toys made in China. Children's costume jewelry laden with cadmium, toys coated with lead, and BPA leaking from sippy cups.

Shiny, plastic things have foiled even my most noble attempts to furnish a green toy wonderland. Just try finding the equivalent of a wooden Exersaucer.

We don't want to deprive our children of the joys of toys, but we're desperately afraid of what permanent effects may be leaching from temporary fun.

Should we really just limit our child's toys to organic corn husks and wooden sticks?

Comedian Lisa Landry avoids plastic toys and anything manufactured overseas—leaving her options pretty slim.

❝ *When he was young, my baby had all wooden toys. We didn't have anything from China in our house, which sucks, because there's nothing made in America, so the kid has the most boring toys possible.* ❞

For Elizabeth, the toys' origin and materials matter less than their coating. She says she doesn't mind plastic toys, finding them lighter and easier to play with than wooden ones, but she worries about the lead content in the paint and the cadmium levels in children's jewelry.

❝ *Especially that funny-looking shiny jewelry, which of course is the stuff my daughter loves. After the initial high, I try to get her to forget about it if I suspect any danger. Many times, that worked, but now that she's five, I have a more difficult time.* ❞

When it comes to toys, having older children is both a blessing and a curse. We don't have to worry as much about everything being a chew toy. However, we struggle as they become far more opinionated.

Mom Hilary said she loosened up as her children got older and stopped putting things in their mouths all the time.

❝ *Then my four-and-a-half-year-old son turned around and chewed through a plastic-encased magnet, so what do I know.* ❞

Carolyn said one morning she came downstairs to find her six-year-old digging in a box of organic cereal, making a huge mess.

❝ *She wanted to know where the toy was.* ❞

Corina says her house overflows with toys supposedly designed to help her son have fun and reach his next milestones.

❝ *I think I'm doing him a favor by getting him the newest and the best things. But then news stories come out almost daily about toxins or un-*

safe materials. After checking the dates and countries of origin on my son's favorite die-cast cars, I threw them out because I was afraid of lead paint. You can't even give the toys away because they may be poisonous. You just have to chalk them up as a loss, dry your kid's tears, and get the next hot thing—after checking the label, of course. **"**

Corina's frustration underlines the fact that while we try to make the best choices as consumers, we also need to lean on our government to make sure they do a better job protecting us from these things. Rick Smith, author of *Slow Death by Rubber Duck: The Secret Danger of Everyday Things* and *Toxin Toxout*, cites labeling requirements as one of the biggest challenges for consumers.

" *You shouldn't have to be a rocket scientist or chemical engineer to shop for toys for your kids. You can be the most active, engaged, savvy consumer in the world, but if you don't have proper labeling on products, you can't tell what you're looking at.* **"**

This is why most scrupulous manufacturers label the absence of phthalates and BPA, Smith says. With strong links to breast and prostate cancer and reproductive abnormalities in little boys, phthalates may be as dangerous as they are difficult to spell.

Smith says phthalates are arguably more common in kids' toys than BPA. Until very recently, most things soft and squishy—i.e., the illustrious rubber duck—would contain phthalates to some level. And if it doesn't say "no phthalates," it probably contains them.

Abby Sher, author of *Amen, Amen, Amen: Memoir of a Girl Who Couldn't Stop Praying (Among Other Things)*, says every time she learns about a dangerous chemical or toxic toy, she feels guilt for having exposed her kids—then tries to trash the stuff, and usually gets caught.

" *The hardest part is hearing about recalls and alerts and fighting back the demons that say I've already caused my children irreparable harm and horns.* **"**

Last spring, my five-year-old and I had planned a special project to share with his preschool friends. The school agreed to set aside a time for me to come do a short presentation on "upcycling" with a fun hands-on project—recycling broken old crayons into new, fun-shaped crayons.

What a treat it would be to teach the kids a great way to recycle and make a cool craft at the same time. For weeks, we collected broken crayons from families, and Sam spread the word that, "Thursday will be a special project with my mommy!" Even the blackboard in the preschool entrance read, "Thursday is Crayon Day!" We were stoked.

Wednesday afternoon, just after I packed up everything I would need for the following day, I opened my laptop to see a steady stream of images and explanation marks on my Facebook feed:

Deadly Asbestos Found in Four Brands of Crayons!
Shocking New Report Finds Asbestos in Kids' Crayons!

And this wasn't some urban-legend stuff. These were legitimate studies done by trusted organization Environmental Working Group. CNN covered the story. It was very real.

Reading the reports, I was naturally appalled—but sadly, not surprised—that crayons could contain actual poison. And though the info frightened me, I would still probably let my kids color with whatever crayons they received at a restaurant or in their goody bags (typically one of the only goody bag items I don't throw out).

But I was about to present a project to a classroom of children where we literally *cook asbestos* and then they go home to tell their parents how they would like to do this on a regular basis.

I had already collected the crayons, and there was a good chance some of them would test positive for asbestos. So it seemed like melting them couldn't be a great idea.

Monona Rossol, chemist and author of *The Artist's Complete Health & Safety Guide*, says if encaustics embedded in wax are fused by heat, the wax converts into airborne emissions and toxic pigments can fume into the air.

❝ *Heating crayons causes problems from the decomposition of the wax and the organic pigments. The asbestos is part of that white bloom you see on the surface of old crayons, migrated to the surface. The fate of the asbestos during heating and torching is unknown.* ❞

So what do I do now that I've promised a bunch of children I would essentially turn their art room/lunchroom into what now feels to me like a meth lab?

First, panic. Second, cry. Third, ask everyone on the internet what they would do.

Some suggest scrapping the project altogether—Rossol, for one, does not recommend melting *any* crayons, asbestos or not.

Others said "screw it" and teach the kids how to burn poison over an open flame. But the most rational minds helped me to find a solution better than trying to create an incredibly lame project where we just glue broken crayons to paper and call it a mosaic.

Sort through the collected crayons and cherry-pick only those that can be identified as Crayola, a made-in-the-USA brand that does not contain asbestos. Sadly, this means I also have to discard any "naked crayons."

Ask the school if I can send a note home in the children's cubbies about what we did, how to replicate the project, and why they should only use Crayola.

Fortunately, everyone was receptive to crayon sorting and accepting this new information along with the learning experience. For any children who asked, I simply explained that some crayons don't melt well—which is also entirely true.

It seems like even the most innocuous of toys causes enough concern to raise red flags at a national level. But despite lead and cadmium in dollar-store trinkets, PVCs in grab machine toys, and even, yes, asbestos in crayons, goody bags continue to overflow with junk from discount importers and retailers.

But it shouldn't be up to the parents to have to fight the local bounce-house party purveyor about their in-house goody bags.

In 1976, The Toxic Substances Control Act (TSCA) approved more than 60,000 existing chemicals used in everyday products, only 200 of which had been tested for safety. More than 80,000 chemicals have been put on the market and made available for use in the four decades since, and the EPA has required very few of these to be tested for their impact on human health and the environment.

This makes it difficult for consumers to find the information they need to identify which chemicals are safe. Instead of requiring chemical manufacturers to demonstrate their products are harmless before they go into use, the law says the government has to prove actual harm in order to control or replace a dangerous chemical.

The Safer Chemicals, Healthy Families coalition spent years calling for an overhaul of TSCA based on the law's inability to protect the health of the American public from exposure to harmful chemicals. Finally, in June 2016, after much lobbying, advocacy, and debate among legislators, the final TSCA reform bill made it to the President's desk.

While it is mostly a victory, Andy Igrejas, director of Safer Chemicals, Healthy Families, said in a press statement that it is not without some serious flaws.

❛❛ *The reform of TSCA gives EPA important new authorities to tackle the problem of toxic chemicals. For the first time, there are also enforceable deadlines and schedules for EPA work on chemicals as well as dedicated funding from fees paid by industry. The pace of change will be slow, however. There are some unnecessary activities required that will divert resources and there are some loopholes in the law. State authority is unduly infringed under the bill, but enough is preserved that states can still take the lead in public health interventions for many, if not most, chemicals.* ❜❜ [1]

This long-fought-for TSCA reform is more limited than environmental and health advocates had hoped for, but it is still meaningful in its protection and a step in the right direction.

Meanwhile, though "Made in the USA" is a label that brings some solace to consumers, it is increasingly difficult to find and not even a sure sign of safer ingredients or practices.

Igrejas says that with most consumer products now being made overseas, there isn't that much evidence to say they are always worse, but it can call into question the rigorousness of the specifications and quality control.

66 *The more the supply chain stretches overseas, the more likely that companies don't know what is in their own product.* **99**

Ironically, though, with higher standards in Europe, products from the EU are often the most safety controlled. And the level of scrutiny in supply chains is growing, thanks in part to Safer Chemicals, Healthy Families and its Mind the Store Campaign, which challenges retailers to restrict chemicals in their supply chains.

In 2015 alone, public campaigns have led to victories, including: Ashley Furniture, the nation's largest furniture retailer, announcing a timeframe for eliminating toxic flame retardants in furniture; Walgreens committing to developing a chemicals policy; Home Depot and Lowe's phasing out added phthalates in flooring by the end of the year; and Walmart and Target both making meaningful progress to implement and expand their chemicals policies.

Unfortunately, no unified label exists to show true chemical safety in toys. However, if a company makes claims about what is *not* in their products, it's in their interest to be able to back them up.

The good news is the scrutiny of toys has increased since the Consumer Product Safety Improvement Act of 2008, at least regarding chemicals like lead, cadmium, and phthalates. But that doesn't mean dollar-store trinkets are safe to chew on, with independent studies still finding high levels of phthalates in bath toys and barrettes.[2]

And that doesn't even cover the low quality and landfill impact of these "cheap thrills."

Mom Carissa is frustrated every time she receives a "surprise box" full of candy and toys from her well-meaning in-laws.

❝ *The cheap toys rarely capture imagination or are durable enough to last very long and inevitably end up being thrown out or donated.* ❞

My own husband recently came home from watching football at a friend's house with a huge Disney suitcase full of hand-me-downs that his well-meaning friend gave him for our two-year-old. We didn't know its contents and made the mistake of opening it in front of the kids. You would have thought I had opened one of those cans that snakes jump out of: dozens of Mardi Gras beads, cheap princess toys, costumes, glitter, and tiaras. My daughter went wild, and I was trying to control my heart palpitations. I threw the worst stuff out when she turned away, but most of it is now part of my life.

Many parents are adept at making goody-bag trinkets and toys "disappear." Some also do big cleanouts and donations in advance of birthdays and holiday season—out with the old junk and in with the new.

Suzan wishes she had more control over the toys her son receives, but realizes she has to choose her battles carefully.

❝ *I think people will buy whatever is convenient to them not really caring whether the toy is harmful or inappropriate to the child. I just throw away cheap, junky toys if we inadvertently get some. I don't believe in donating them because why give some other kid a toxic toy?* ❞

Sharon believes a "cheap, junky toy" can create its own lesson in sustainability.

❝ *I usually let my kids keep toys in goody bags for a few days—and then they fall apart. When this happens, I try to make a note to my six-year-old about how the junky toy fell apart after a day and how these are not the kind of toys we want to buy.* ❞

But if the newest toys are the safest, does that take the eco-savvy out of shopping secondhand or enjoying heirloom toys?

Personally, unless you are buying something to teethe on, I wouldn't give up used or older toys.

My Fisher Price and Playskool toys from the '70s and '80s were made in the USA. Nothing shone, sparkled, or required batteries. And back then, manufacturers used fewer chemicals or plastic varieties.

And as for more modern secondhand toys, I just stick to the same basic guidelines and Google for product recalls. Another plus side of older toys is that they've had a while to off-gas any volatile organic compounds.

But Melodie, a mother of four, says while she used to see second-hand shopping as the answer to the toy problem, she has gained a new perspective. She believes the goal shouldn't just be to reduce spending and the demand for new toys, but to use toys as a way to teach children about a broader sense of stewardship.

❝ *All of these cheaply made toys result in piles of unloved, frequently broken items. The toy box becomes not a place to keep toys safe but to ensure toys are broken. How can I teach my children to value what they have, and to value repairing above discarding, when they have too many toys to count, and repairing the broken ones is so difficult? Many toys are sold with the idea that they will be in a landfill in a year's time.* ❞

Melodie says she does go the used toy route because she's found that if a toy has made it through its first life in another home, it's that much more likely to make it through life in theirs.

❝ *But we are more open to new toys from companies that are willing to stand by their products and help us to fix them if they should break. Keeping our focus on this issue has had the added benefit of reducing our consumption of toys that are worse for the environment without us having to think much about that side of things. Turns out that toy companies that are trying to make toys that last are also less prone to making toys that are chemical-laden or entirely made of synthetic materials.* ❞

Actress Alysia Reiner ("Orange is the New Black") echoes the sentiment that creativity and imagination are key and we should encourage our children to do more with less.

❝ *When Liv was younger and put everything in her mouth, I was very particular about everything and freaked about all plastics entering the house. Now that she is six, I just try to make it about creativity—reusing boxes and toilet paper rolls so we are both recycling and reusing and also making, not wasting. We take old pajamas and make our own dolls or clothes or blankets for my old dollhouse. I find if I keep the focus on creating, she has less desire for Dora, Barbie, Disney princesses—she wants to be her own hero.* **❞**

Questionable trinkets are unavoidable, popping up everywhere from the dentist's office to your great aunt's purse. We can hide objects, toss things, and steer clear of the toy store, but it sounds like the best strategy is to teach our children the true value of playthings. Sure, they will want to collect all the Shopkins and complain that everyone else has Bratz dolls, but opportunities to play with things not of our choosing will present themselves no matter what. So we can set our own boundaries and arm ourselves with the knowledge that a dearth of cheap plastic toys does not make them *deprived*. Our children will find much more joy in the long run from learning to care for special things, using their imaginations, and being resourceful.

Just remember, no matter how hard you try, it's only a matter of time before you will step on a Lego block.

T I P S for the Toy Box

✔ Shopping for sustainably made, well-crafted toys can pay for itself in longevity and ease toxicity concerns.

✔ Secondhand toys can be great for wallets and landfills, but be sure to check for recalls and be wary of anything that sets off the chemical alarm (soft, squishy plastic; shiny, metallic glow; so cheaply made you can't believe it survived this long).

✔ When checking out plastic toys, look for the same numbers you probably check for recycling. Numbers 1, 2, 4, and 5 are the least problematic and, not so coincidentally, the easiest to recycle. Stay away from numbers 3, 6, and 7; they may leach dangerous chemicals and inevitably end up in landfills anyway.

✔ My personal rule of thumb is to avoid anything metallic or shiny that may be painted with lead or cadmium, anything made of soft, squishy plastic (think cereal box crawlers), and anything with fragrance, like scratch-and-sniff stickers. I also don't trust anything that bursts out of a piñata or emerges from a plastic egg.

✔ Sign up for action alerts from saferchemicals.org and healthystuff.org to advocate for stricter regulation of toxic chemicals in toys and other consumer products. You can also check safer product shopping guides at sites like thesoftlanding.com.

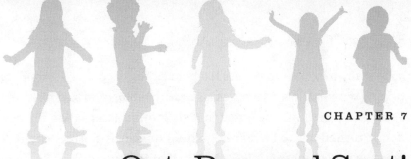

CHAPTER 7

Out, Damned Spot!

Baking Soda Versus the Superbug

MY FIRST PREGNANCY coincided with the 2009 Swine Flu scare.

First, it just affected people in Mexico. Then, the potentially deadly virus reached the States where, as the media made it seem, it was spreading faster than a YouTube video of a cat playing the keyboard.

After a couple months of nightly news reports and paper face masks, the flu waned with relatively minimal casualties. It wasn't until around the time I gave birth that the fall flu season brought with it the second wave of swine flu—or H1N1, as it became better known, to prevent the slaughter of innocent pigs—with a certified pandemic and rising death toll.

Everyone was strongly urged to get vaccinated, though the elusive shots were harder to come by than a spot in a New York City preschool. When the vaccines did start to trickle in, they were only available for pregnant women, and OB/GYN offices had strict orders not to "waste" their dosages on new mothers with highly susceptible infants.

I kept hearing horror stories about babies in intensive care with the H1N1 virus, barely being kept alive on ventilators. But even when the vaccine would become more widely available, it was not meant for babies younger than six months old.

Like hordes of other nervous new mothers, I flocked to message boards, desperate to find a doctor who would at least vaccinate me so that my baby would be less likely to suffer exposure. I ended up bribing a pediatrician 30 miles away with a box of mixed nuts and a sob story. (It should be noted that six months later, when the epidemic turned out to be more of a mild nuisance, doctors couldn't give the vaccines away—less than half of the 229 million doses of vaccine were used.[1])

In the meantime, people across the country cancelled playdates, lathered themselves in hand sanitizer, and avoided sick people like, well, the plague. Doctors' office waiting rooms banned magazines for fear of spreading germs via cardboard perfume sample.

Afraid that my organic peppermint and castile soap wouldn't do the trick, I kept a bottle of hand sanitizer right by the door, asking all visitors to thoroughly cleanse before thinking about touching the baby. Meticulously swathed in the potent salve, we kept easy-access hand sanitizers in our pockets and our purses. Motion detection dispensers were on the walls of every office building and next to every elevator. We moms even rubbed it on our babies' hands after they—God forbid—touched another child's toy.

Imagine our surprise when we heard the news that several toddlers were treated for alcohol poisoning after licking their sanitized hands. The very thing we used to protect our children from illness was getting them more hammered than we were on our prom nights.

The modern mother is forced to walk a fine line between disinfecting and intoxicating. For every warning of food-borne illness and careful hand washing, we are alerted to the hazards of bleach and alcohol.

How do we keep our homes safe and relatively bacteria free without putting our children in a bubble?

Striving for an unreachable standard of sterile is a dangerous high-wire act for moms who want the best for their kids, says Sandra, a West Coast mother of two.

66 *What's more important? Sanitary or safe? Why not just give up on being sterile all together? I have thought for a while that the hand sanitizers are really drying and smell fumy. They can't be good to breathe or*

for little hands, and they seem really unnecessary to me. Why not just wash your hands using a nontoxic hand soap and call it a wrap? 99

Michele Beschen, host of *b. organic with Michele Beschen* on PBS, says she believes a little dirt is "good for us" and is more concerned with letting in fresh air than air fresheners.

66 *I want a vibrant home that embraces nature rather than neurosis. I'm not the type of person that freaks out if someone sneezes, wheezes, and hacks all over me and then expects to get sick myself. At our house, we rarely, if ever, fall ill to the flu or colds. We're not scrubbing down shopping carts or rubbing ourselves down with hand sanitizer at every turn. I'm more of an advocate of a healthy home—a home filled with fresh air, green plants, and surfaces that are easy to keep clean like hard surface floors and wood furnishings.* 99

Philadelphia NBC 10 news anchor and mother Denise Nakano also avoids anything that says "antibacterial."

66 *There are so many options on store shelves, including many products labeled antibacterial. I tend to avoid them and go with regular soap. I don't want to overdo it and I certainly don't want to create super germs through the use of antibacterial soaps.* 99

Leslie says she thinks she's doing her family a favor by being a slacker in the cleaning department.

66 *My daughter's teacher noticed that when all the kids had hand sanitizers at their cubbies, the floor tiles were discolored where the sanitizer had dripped. Increasingly, studies show that farm kids (raised, ostensibly, with more exposure to pathogens, etc.) have incredible immune systems compared to their urban counterparts.[2] Exposure to germs when they're that young creates strong immune systems. It's harder to fight an enemy you've never encountered.* 99

Leslie refers to "The Hygiene Hypothesis," a theory first proposed in the late '80s to explain why allergic diseases were less common in children from larger families (of disease-spreading siblings).[3] This hypothesis suggests that extremely clean household environments derail a baby's immune response by failing to provide the necessary exposure to germs required to "educate" the immune system to launch its defense responses. Instead, the baby's defense responses end up being so inadequate that they actually contribute to the development of asthma.[4]

Mom Lori also doesn't see the point in carrying Purell wherever she goes.

66 *I've read research about how they're not effective and sometimes counterproductive in terms of killing germs. I am the opposite of a germaphobe though. I'm one of those people who would roll my daughter in the mud because it's good for her immune system. But I also had pinworms more than once as a child, so…* 99

Many squirts of sanitizer later, my son has yet to be face down after a long night of karaoke and drunk-dialing exes. But according to Dr. Ronald Stram, director and founder of the Stram Center for Integrative Medicine in Delmar, NY, getting drunk is not the problem with sanitizers.

As long as the kids aren't chugging from the bottle, there is generally too little alcohol left on their hands, especially since it will mostly evaporate, he said. The real issue lies more with Stram's faith in the hygiene hypothesis. He cites the abundance of MRSA skin infections as the possible result of overuse of antibacterial skin cleansers.

66 *The hygiene hypothesis has significant merit. Exposure to harmless bacteria or viruses instills an immune surveillance system capable of responding better to harmful bugs. The overuse of antibiotics tends to increase the likelihood of continued infections because our innate defense system has been compromised.* 99

Stram also notes that the health risk of "superbugs" is actually a valid concern. He says between the use of triclosan—the most popular antibacterial agent in cleansers—and antibiotics in non-bacterial-related (viral) illnesses, superbugs are becoming a health risk.

Which puts the ball of this debate back into the courts of the slightly "dirtier" contingency. But Stram does not advocate letting all hell break loose in your living room. This is, happily, an area where middle ground is just fine.

According to Stram, the ideal scenario for optimum health should actually give moms a sigh of relief. We are right to demand proper hand washing before dinner, but we can also ease up on sanitizing that Lego.

66 *I would recommend not cleaning toys consistently with disinfectants. You want to raise the immune system of the individual by exposure, as long as it's done in a relatively safe way where you're maintaining good hygiene habits. In terms of being obsessive about clean toys and surfaces, I don't think that is beneficial for the people or the environment.* 99

In this vein, moms like Janice say they try to simplify and take a DIY attitude, tolerating more dirt and cleaning with fewer products. Though she does admit to one bathroom that only seems to respond to the caustic, bleachy stuff, she generally sticks to vinegar, water, and microfiber towels.

66 *Hand sanitizer is a last resort, a particularly nasty diaper change in the park or only because I used a porta-potty kind of solution.* 99

Janice is part of the growing trend of people going back to the good old days of castile soap, baking soda, vinegar, and essential oils. Actress Kaitlin Olson ("It's Always Sunny in Philadelphia") makes her own all-purpose house cleaner with simple ingredients.

66 *It sounds super irritating, but it only takes 30 seconds. And I save a ton of money on cleaning products.* 99

The DIY moms can be confident in Stram's encouraging the use of simple, cheap, natural cleaners like vinegar.

66 *Vinegar creates an unfriendly acidic environment that doesn't support most bacterial and fungal growth. It does not kill bugs, which is probably ecologically better, because bugs don't become resistant in this environment but do learn to be stronger or better with continued use of antibiotics.* 99

And he says worries about flu bugs easily swimming around in salad dressing are likely unfounded. These little critters need to exist in quantity to inoculate to the point where they cause disease.

66 *If you're creating an environment where replication of the bug is not favorable, then you're essentially using an ecologically friendly way of getting rid of your enemies. It doesn't kill them per se, but it creates an environment where they just die off.* 99

So in being eco-friendly with our cleaners, apparently we aren't just treading humanely on the planet. Some might say we are creating good karma by treading lightly among those very smallest of living things—bacteria. But if you aren't the type to gently lead a spider out your window, you certainly don't have to buy into that.

Sometimes it becomes a matter of principle for mothers, frustrated by companies' lack of concern, consistency, and disclosure.

Gina, a mother of two, says she is even more concerned about the ingredients in cleaning products than food, because they give the idea of a thing being "clean," but in reality, they could be loaded with dangerous toxins.

66 *So when you go about your life, your kids may be putting food, pacifiers, utensils, chew toys, and other items in their mouth or on their skin along with those toxins—unless you make safe choices. I'm especially concerned with dishwashing liquids and laundry detergent.* 99

Supermodel Emme says she is also concerned about what's in the ingredients of conventional cleaning products.

66 *I have lack of faith that big corporate conventional product companies are taking the time to look out for my family's health. I go to great*

lengths to find the right eco-friendly and natural product that will do just as good a job if not better than a conventional brand. "

Erin Switalski is the executive director of Women's Voices for the Earth. For more than 20 years, this women's health nonprofit has helped lead the fight to disclose toxic ingredients in cleaning products, fragrances, cosmetics, and feminine hygiene products. Women's Voices focuses specifically on cancer-causing chemicals that directly and disproportionately impact women's health. Its campaigns have challenged such chemical giants as SC Johnson and Son, Procter & Gamble, the Clorox Company, and more.

Switalski says she has seen some leading manufacturers phase out a number of harmful chemicals, including phthalates, synthetic musks, glycol ethers, triclosan, and 1,4-dioxane. But the main problem is we still don't have full ingredient disclosure. The words "fragrance" or "parfum" on a product label represents an undisclosed mixture of various scent chemicals.

" *We also have no guarantee that companies won't find a new chemical of concern to add to their products. We need companies to have fully transparent chemical-screening processes. We need to know they are making sure new ingredients and products are safe.* "

It's difficult for the average consumer to avoid confusion with cleaning and personal care products, but the first thing to do is to make sure you buy products with the full ingredients on the label.

There are a few new but growing third-party certifications for consumer products, including "Green Seal," the EPA's "Safer Choices," and Environmental Working Group's "EWG Verified." There's also a new certification process for products launched by a nonprofit called Nontoxic Certified. Their "MADE SAFE" screening process determines that all the raw ingredients used to make a product are deemed safe and have been vetted by an independent third party. But until these new labels become mainstream, consumers can also check the ratings of cleaning and personal care products in the Environmental Working Group's Skin Deep and Cleaners databases.

But why should *we* have to do all this research? Shouldn't companies be required to limit or at least disclose cancer-causing chemicals in their products?

Switalski says there is a very powerful lobby of chemical companies that spends millions of dollars to maintain the status quo.

❝ *The only way to truly break through this is to create a groundswell of consumers calling on companies to make safer products and on Congress to enact health-protective laws. Every person can make a difference by calling a company and demanding safe products or making a call to their senator or representative. Organizations like Women's Voices for the Earth are set up to help consumers make these requests.* ❞

Even products especially designed for babies are not immune to a debatable idea of clean.

In response to consumer pressure, Johnson & Johnson pledged to remove formaldehyde and 1,4-dioxane from its baby products by the end of 2013. Yes, prior to that, formaldehyde was an ingredient in the familiar baby shampoo given to new moms in hospitals across the country. Executives said Johnson & Johnson was responding to a fundamental shift in consumer behavior, as an increasingly informed public demands that companies be more responsive to concerns about product ingredients.[5]

But even as more sustainable, clean, and toxin-free products become available, many parents have vices they can't seem to part with.

The strong, pungent scent of bleach seems to emit olfactory nostalgia for so many parents who can't seem to quit it. Some parents seek—and successfully find—satisfactory sustainable replacements for conventional antiperspirants and hair dye. But just about everyone has a guilty pleasure or two.

Actress Alysia Reiner thought she couldn't live without Crème de la Mer until she weaned herself off with a natural face serum and coconut oil. Jenny in Dallas says she struggles finding a natural conditioner since her hair is fragile from coloring.

66 *Right now, I use a vegan and mostly organic option, but I am sure it's not perfect because I dye my hair bright purple.* **99**

Lori says she rarely wears makeup, but when she does, it's the cheap drugstore variety.

66 *I tend to be much more careful about the things that will impact my daughter than I am with my own things.* **99**

Latoya is concerned about her teenage daughter's allergies and asthma, as she is currently lured to questionable cosmetics.

66 *When my daughter first started wearing makeup a friend had encouraged her to get cheap makeup from the dollar store.* **99**

The good news is we can wean ourselves off some of our more un-eco-friendly addictions as more effective and accessible non-toxic alternatives come to market. Jessica Alba's Honest Company has mainstreamed a better diaper cream, while BeautyCounter has adopted the multilevel-marketing model for nontoxic beauty products. Free sites like kind-eye.com offer safer product matching for consumers who don't think they can give up their favorite eyeliner.

We can be clean and pretty while being safe and conscious at the same time. Less isn't just more when making up your face, but also when you're looking at ingredient lists. Let's use products that leave us free to lick our lips, lick our fingers, and lick our plates clean when no one is watching.

T I P S for Safer Cleaning

✔ Hygiene is important. Compulsive scrubbing with anti-bacterial products is not. Good old-fashioned hand washing with plain soap and water is your best bet.

✔ Hand sanitizer probably won't give you alcohol poisoning. But overuse could possibly do more harm than good. And when the situation calls for sanitizer, try a more natural brand like CleanWell.

✔ Vinegar works for more than low-calorie salad dressing. I'm also a huge fan of certain essential oils, which are effective antimicrobials.[6]

✔ When it comes to cleaning and personal care products, a handful of third-party certifications exist but nothing is streamlined or mandated. Without regulation, it's best to become acquainted with EWG's online databases or shop stores that do the research for you, like spiritbeautylounge .com, capbeauty.com, and thedetoxmarket.com.

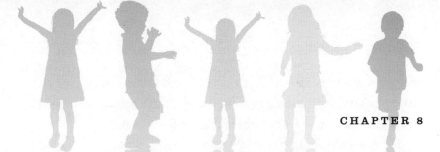

CHAPTER 8

A Better Home Through Chemistry?

Or, Is My Kitchen Going to Kill Me?

I AM AFRAID of my kitchen.

I enjoy cooking, and I unquestionably enjoy eating. And every time I come home with a new vegetable share from my CSA or even a well-timed Fresh Direct delivery, I take pleasure in finding new recipes that I know at least three out of the four of us will enjoy.

The problem is I am completely terrified that my cookware will kill me.

I've known for some time I will probably die a slow death from the few plastic remnants in my kitchen. The culprits are hard to avoid: old plastic containers that have gone through the heat cycle on the dishwasher a million times and those BPA-free bottles that may actually be made with something just as toxic.

I've baked bread in a chipped nonstick breadmaker and sautéed on scratched up "eco-friendly" nonstick cookware I suspect might have qualities just as worrisome as any other chemically coated pan.

Or maybe I'll die by homemade pipe bomb, as could have easily happened when a perfectly fine-seeming piece of Pyrex glassware inexplicably and violently shattered as I took it out of the oven. I later learned that, several years ago, good old American Pyrex decided to use a less temperature-resistant (and cheaper) form of glass.[1] Now I literally have to screw up courage any time I take a dish in or out of the oven. And forget the gas stove—I've always been convinced that thing is gonna blow from an errant crumb in the burner.

My environmentally irresponsible Keurig was also recalled for spewing hot liquid and burning several customers.[2] I once absent-mindedly stuck my finger in a hand blender while making pesto and had to get stitches.

Maybe we were better off before the advent of fire, and I'd feel safer sticking to nuts and berries. Except that everyone I know is allergic to nuts. And it's impossible to find organic berries in the winter.

And I'm not the only one tearing up my kitchen.

Suzan, a mother of a seven-year-old, joins the thousands of people throwing out their expensive sets of nonstick pots and pans.

  " *My husband wasn't too happy about it, but it had to be done.* **"**

If you registered for your wedding gifts in the past 50 years, you probably have a few nonstick metal pans coated with a synthetic polymer commonly known as Teflon. There is peer-reviewed research—as well as sad anecdotal evidence—that the toxic fumes from the Teflon chemical released from pots and pans at high temperatures are actually notorious for killing pet birds.[3] Additionally, studies link chemicals in the Teflon family with various adverse health and environmental effects.[4]

Dawn Lerman, author of *My Fat Dad: A Memoir of Food, Love and Family, with Recipes*, says she got rid of all her Teflon pans and replaced them with some of the nonstick pans on the market making safer "green" and "eco" claims.

  " *I buy the 'eco-pans,' but every couple months when they get scratched up, I no longer trust them so I replace them. But I guess that's not doing the landfills any favors.* **"**

Plastic has plagued parents since we learned about its tendency to leach and degrade into our food and beverages.

Amy Wilson, actress and author of *When Did I Get Like This?*, says after deliberating the inconsistent media messaging about the safety of BPA in plastic, the final verdict taught her a lesson about "not being too quick to dismiss the voices that are out front on such issues as kooks, or fringe, or obsessing about nothing."

❝ *There were plenty of people saying BPA was dangerous when my baby was born seven years ago, but they were pooh-poohed, and any mother who was tossing out the plastic sippy cups back in 2003 would have had many eyes rolled at her behind her back. Now, it turns out I should have been concerned all this time and thrown out all that stuff years ago when I first heard about it. I want to be a calm, non-overthinking mom, but the next time I hear about something like this, I'll listen the first time.* **❞**

Once upon a time, plastics were supposed to completely improve our quality of life. If a plastic incubator can save a baby's life, should we be prejudiced against all better living through chemistry?

Because no labeling requirements exist, it's hard to say when chemicals like phthalates and bisphenol A (BPA) first came into use as a common component of consumer products. But in the '70s and '80s (shortly after Mr. McGuire's prediction in *The Graduate*) there was a noticeable trend upward in the use of plastics in everyday life.

In 2007, reports from the National Institutes of Health and the US National Toxicology Program announced "some concern" about BPA's effects on fetal and infant brain development and behavior.[5] "BPA" soon became a scary buzzword, leaving parents ransacking their cabinets.

Then in February 2011, a widely reported study titled "Most Plastic Products Release Estrogenic Chemicals" created concern that even BPA- and phthalate-free plastics could potentially leak carcinogens and hormones.[6] The study found that more than 70 percent of the plastic food and beverage containers tested contained chemicals that acted like estrogen—and that was *before* exposure to heat, light, or general wear.

It was enough to make parents want to put the lid on all plastic containers and swap to solely glass and stainless steel. But even the rubber-coated Duralex plastic glasses can shatter into a thousand pieces when thrown by an irate toddler. Were we being forced to choose between shards of glass underfoot now or precocious puberty later?

Dr. Alan Greene, pediatrician and author of *Raising Baby Green: The Earth-Friendly Guide to Pregnancy, Childbirth, and Baby Care*, assures us that we can still use some plastics without great risk. And certainly, some plastics are safer than others.

Greene suggests going with sounder plastics like numbers 2, 4, and 5. He also recommends sticking with companies that seriously think about these issues and not just take out BPA because it's a buzz item right now. He also notes that high heat should continue to be avoided and plastics should be replaced when there is noticeable wear and tear.

Beyond concerns about plastics, we hear the dangers of flame retardants in our furniture, car seats, and crib mattresses. Studies have linked various flame retardants to thyroid disruption, memory and learning problems, delayed mental and physical development, lower IQ, advanced puberty and reduced fertility, and cancer.[7]

All these chemical concerns have actually stopped mom Carissa from buying some new things.

66 *I've wanted a new couch for years, but I know the one I have now has just about finished off-gassing and a new would be more toxic.* 99

The good news is, thanks to a key policy change in California fire safety standards, mainstream furniture manufacturers like Pottery Barn and IKEA now produce sofas and sectionals without flame-retardant chemicals. All IKEA couches manufactured after January 1, 2015, are made without chemical flame-retardants, and West Elm, Pottery Barn, and Crate & Barrel will follow suit.

If you choose to use older furniture or something secondhand, learn as much as you can about the product's origin—when and where it was made and by whom, suggests Megan Boyle, editorial director of Healthy Child Healthy World and the Environmental Working Group.

❝ *Products have changed over the years as new chemicals have entered the marketplace and others have been banned. Workmanship and quality materials matter. Secondhand furniture made of solid, real wood can be a better choice than the particleboard in use today.* ❞

But if you are a fan of true vintage like me, the biggest chemical concern is old paint that may contain lead.

As the second year of my son's life yielded increased mobility, I realized it takes a child's-eye-view to spot a dreaded microscopic enemy even the most vigilant mother had yet to catch: crumbling lead paint under the back door.

I felt confident the remnants of 60-year-old paint were safely contained under several coats of low-VOC paint. But I didn't check the most prevalent, and often neglected, areas for the use of lead paint in homes built before 1978—door and window frames.

A visit from a lead abatement specialist cited not only the possibility of lead in my home's structure but also a serious critique of my penchant for antique furniture. I thought shabby chic was eco-stylish, not potentially dangerous? But there it was—rooms full of my ancestors' paint-chipped drawers and lovingly broken-down flea market finds, all among my son's favorite items to open, close, examine, and crawl under. Add in his extraordinary keen eye for finding every speck of dirt to try out on his tongue—not helped by the fact that children are attracted to lead because it actually tastes *sweet*.

Years later during a room remodel, construction workers used a wet saw to cut tile on my deck, spraying my blossoming blueberry and basil plants with a coating of white powder. That's when I learned that even *new tile* can contain lead, as it is still allowed in ceramic glazes. This fact forced me to not only thoroughly wash the plants but replant them as well.

With the American Academy of Pediatrics recommending children be tested for lead twice before age three, many parents have been shocked by the results—and the realization that lead is still a pervasive problem.

Mom Rachel had the foresight to check areas of her older home using a store-bought lead test. After finding positive results around the windowsills, she hired certified lead painters to mitigate the situation.

   66 *Fortunately, the pediatrician tested the kids for lead and the tests came back negative. But I know another mom who has lead in her house and her son's levels were a little high. Maybe it is a coincidence, but he has a weird twitch and behavior problems at school. I sometimes wonder if he has some of the symptoms of lead exposure.* 99

Tamara Rubin, a mother of four in Portland, OR, founded Lead Safe America Foundation (LSAF) in 2011 after years of volunteer advocacy work following the lead poisoning of two of her children in 2005. Her children's lead levels skyrocketed after negligent contractors used illegal practices to remove exterior paint from her older home. LSAF offers emergency intervention and support to families whose children have been diagnosed as positive for lead in their blood.

If your house was built before 1980, Tamara recommends getting a professional hazard assessment, which can range from free for qualifying homeowners in select cities to up to $2,000. If a professional assessment is not available, order an easy-to-use home lead test kit for free at leadsafeamerica.org. And if any lead is found, always hire EPA-RRP certified contractors.

I know—it's enough to make you want to go live in a hut.

But without a hand-built log cabin on the horizon, moms like Kristen are left to fret over home renovations.

   66 *I'm worried about paint fumes, the stains we used on our hardwoods when they get refinished, and the new carpeting we just put over the asbestos floor in our basement.* 99

Rick Smith, author of *Slow Death by Rubber Duck* and *Toxin Toxout*, says the good news is that by being a little more careful with what you use and buy, you can dramatically lower levels of these chemicals in your body—sometimes within in a matter of hours. Our bodies can quite effectively flush phthalates and BPA out of our systems, offering a detoxifying reprieve similar to quitting smoking.

Unfortunately, he says, that quick effect doesn't apply to all chemicals—Teflon, found in things like cookware and stain repellent, and flame retardants, found in clothing and upholstery, linger in your body, and in some cases you never get rid of them.[8]

Of course, it would be cumbersome and exhausting to go through every potential toxin in every room with a fine toothcomb. But it's a good idea to take a look at your home and make changes that are realistic and plausible.

You can start by replacing or repairing anything that is concernedly worn (scratched pans, chipped paints, warped plastic) and by carefully considering any new purchases.

We must be brave and live in the 21st century. Stir those pots with some faith that hot oil won't shoot directly into our eyes. Bake those cookies with abandon.

It takes balls to feed a family of four. Balls of stainless steel.

▨▨▨▨ to Detox Your Home

✓ Get rid of anything with a strong fragrance or chemical smell—a likely sign of endocrine-disrupting phthalates. Common culprits: plastic shower curtains, plug-in air fresheners, and most scented candles.

✓ Pare down as much plastic as possible from your kitchen. Don't put heated food in plastic—in fact, don't heat plastic, period.

✓ Healthy Child Healthy World's "9 Steps to a Healthier Kitchen" contains important—albeit slightly scary—information, including the three types of cookware least likely to kill you (unless you drop them on your head): cast iron, enameled cast iron (my favorite), and stainless steel.

✓ Avoid anything labeled as "nonstick" or "stain repellent," often a sign of PFCs. Learn how to season a cast iron pan with cooking oil and remove stains with baking soda instead.

✓ A good organic crib mattress starts at $250. I know—it's a lot. I suggest splurging on the mattress and saving on the crib. IKEA cribs have pretty rigorous safety standards and start at $79. It's also easy to find affordable organic cotton sheets at places like Target. Stuck with a traditional mattress? Let your new mattress off-gas outside or in a well-ventilated area for a while before using it and cover it with an organic cotton cover or a natural latex, wool, or cotton mattress topper.

✓ Get a HEPA air purifier. Not only will it help absorb some of the yucky stuff and allergens in the air, it will also make great white noise.

CHAPTER 9

Learning Your
ABCs and PCBs

Can School Be More a Setback
Than a Safe Haven?

CONCERNED ABOUT ELEVATED levels of toxic chemicals in class-room window caulking, supermodel Cindy Crawford pulled her two children out of Malibu High School in 2014. The high school randomly tested ten classrooms for polychlorinated biphenyl (PCBs)—banned from use since 1979 due to their link to cancer and other adverse health conditions—and four were well over the federal limit.

My son's elementary school was built in 1909. I'd venture to guess it wouldn't take too much searching to find asbestos, lead, PCBs, and the skeletons of our nation's forefathers. (The school is just yards from Philadelphia's "Tomb of the Unknown Soldier." Haley Joel Osment would surely see dead people.)

With budget cuts eliminating building upgrades for schools across America, parents like Marissa are concerned about what might be lurking in the walls.

❝ One thing I had to verify was that my kid's preschool was lead-free. The way-too-scary fact is that there are preschools, elementary schools, and high schools in our country still coated with lead-based paint. These toxic environments can cause much more long-term harm than many realize. ❞

Add to this that public and even private schools are mandated to clean with industrial bleach and serve up cheap pink soap teeming with triclosan, a ubiquitous consumer antibacterial already under scrutiny by the Food and Drug Administration (FDA), thanks to recent reports that it can disrupt hormones and promote tumor growth.[1]

Actress Kaitlin Olson ("It's Always Sunny in Philadelphia") says that when her kids first started preschool, she would watch them go wash their hands, barely rinse it off, and then sit down to eat lunch with bubbles still on their hands.

66 I panicked. I don't want to be the irritating mom who starts preaching about triclosan in antibacterial soap and how it's banned in Canada and Europe. But I also don't want my kids eating it! 99

Back-to-school supply lists request antibacterial wipes and hand sanitizers, despite the fact that the FDA admits there is no evidence cleaning with disinfectants is any better at preventing illness than cleaning with regular soap and water.[2]

Traditional disinfectant cleaners often contain chemicals linked to asthma, allergies, and other health concerns. And while the ethyl alcohol in traditional hand sanitizers may not be of major toxicity concern, the undisclosed chemical fragrances in many varieties can be endocrine disruptors.

As most teachers may not be receptive to cleaning with vinegar and water or enforcing a stricter hand-washing regimen, the next best idea is choosing products with more natural active ingredients and phthalate-free formulas. For instance, the active ingredients in CleanWell hand sanitizer and Seventh Generation Wipes are formulations of thyme oil, which the EPA considers to be a minimal risk.

But moms like Suzan are pretty sure most parents won't be bringing in these slightly more expensive, less toxic varieties.

66 I'm concerned about product fumes trapped inside the classrooms. I'm trying to help implement as many healthy and nontoxic products as possible. However, that also takes a lot of money to do, so I try to implement small, reasonable changes. 99

It can feel like a hotbed of toxicity—and unless you choose to homeschool, your options for improvement are limited. And moms like Carolyn are just hoping more parents take notice.

66 *I worry about fumes from dry erase markers and disinfecting wipes on the school supply list, but although I try my darnedest, I can't make other people send healthy alternatives. I know there are people that should care and don't, but there are also people that are trying to make ends meet and may not have the bandwidth or budget to make these choices possible. I like to lead by example but not shame or judge others.* 99

Jennifer Hankey is an Atlanta mother of two who started Healthy Green Schools, an educational school greening program, in 2012.

66 *When I started this program, the majority of people thought I was nuts and we were 'all just fine.' But just by educating one mom at a time, one principal at a time, I now have 35 schools doing the program.* 99

Jennifer started with her daughter's school, making every change she could. She drummed up parents and made them tell the school they cared.

66 *The staff was not excited about it at first. But the director was a strong leader who decided this was here to stay. They loved and embraced the changes so much that they had me speak to a group of schools. When they liked the idea and signed up, Healthy Green Schools was born.* 99

Advocating for change is not always such an easy task, especially when you are dealing with schools funded at the federal level. Jennifer explains that public schools are more difficult for a multitude of reasons.

66 *Generally, the schools are cleaned by huge cleaning contracts that are won by bids, and safer chemicals are not really considered as a factor. Then, many public schools ask parents to purchase the sanitizing wipes and donate them. My attempts to get teachers to ask for safer*

products have not been successful, and I've had more luck having the parent teacher association pay for the safer products and provide them. A strong PTA and parent support is critical as well as a staff meeting explaining why this is so important and how it will impact the students. 99

Jennifer says the key is finding other parents who care. A flyer going around a Houston public school illustrates the power of collaboration by likening one parent to "a fruitcake," three parents to "troublemakers," ten parents as "we'd better listen," and 50 parents as "a powerful organization."

66 *Get a group or committee going, invite more and more parents, educate everyone around you, and build momentum. This is the only way in a public school. In private schools, it can be the same way or can be as simple as one really passionate parent reaching out to the head of school.* 99

I learned that change was possible, but sometimes hard won, when my own children attended a nonprofit preschool that relied on additional fundraising for supplemental income. While it is a progressive school, old habits die hard, and I led an uphill battle with my request to swap conventional apples and berries for organic.

Though I know fresh fruit for snack time is an amenity most preschools sadly don't provide at all (my son occasionally attends an aftercare where he receives a choice of Doritos, Oreos, or Nabisco's Chicken in a Biskit crackers), I thought at least upgrading away from the "dirty dozen" was worth rallying for. I researched produce providers, compared prices, and searched for clever solutions, like becoming a CSA pickup spot for a free weekly box. My attempts were fruitless (pun intended).

But just because I had lost one battle didn't mean the war was over. My push for greener cleaning products was met halfway, with Seventh Generation wipes and CleanWell hand sanitizer becoming welcome mainstays, while harsh conventional cleaners still made appearances in the school bathrooms.

To the credit of persistence and the bottom dollar, I did achieve one victory to make my lasting legacy—the switch to nontoxic, organic sunscreen. I knew from the start the kids were lathered with Coppertone in the summertime and made sure we provided our own alternative sunscreen for my kids. But as reports from Environmental Working Group continued to list Coppertone Water Babies in their "hall of shame," I thought there might be a way to work with a trusted brand and strike a deal.[3]

Would a newer organic sunscreen brand like Goddess Garden provide wholesale prices to a nonprofit preschool? The answer was yes, and the financial benefits were indisputable. Even with Coppertone ordered by the case, the organic brand wholesale prices won out. The administration agreed to give it a shot, and the change was officially made.

Progress is much more difficult at the public school level due to red tape and contracts. With a private school, if you can prove a cost savings, you can often make an airtight case.

But even with public schools, sometimes all you have to do is ask. When my son's kindergarten teacher asked parents to chip in for school supplies, I offered to pay more to get a case of nontoxic wipes and hand sanitizers. But the teacher immediately replied that buying eco-friendly supplies was no problem. I lucked out—but parents like Betsy know it isn't always so simple.

❝ *I often find it so exhausting to be swimming upstream. I'm sick of the sugar at my kids' school—which is more than 90 percent low-income Hispanic. I feel like passing out an article about how half of all America (and an even higher rate for Latinos) is diabetic or pre-diabetic. But I don't. Because I'm annoying enough as it is, making a stink about homework and other educational issues. It's so hard to only pick a few battles.* ❞

Supermodel Emme, mother of a 13-year-old, says she has tried to advocate for progress at her daughter's school, but it's not easy to change a school struggling to get funding for the basics.

❝ I'm hugely concerned that while children are learning, they're breathing in noxious fumes and toxins due to budgets being cut. When you suggest eco-friendly cleaning products or, even bigger, having the school tested for nasty toxins, they think about lost days equaling less pay. ❞

Jennifer Hankey points out that people generally do not like change or to think what they may be doing or using can be harmful. But the food changes are by far the most difficult—getting junk foods out of the classroom in particular.

❝ This seems to meet deep resentment and resistance even with the stunning numbers of obesity in our schools. But in general, I find the majority of parents and teachers are interested in healthy options once they are told the harmful effects of the foods and products they use. ❞

Jennifer says the key is presenting solutions.

❝ When my children have been in schools that are not open to change, I provide all the soaps, sanitizers, and nontoxic wipes for the year. That may not be an option for everyone. Try to get other moms in your classroom to go in with you. Offer to provide non-food rewards for the classroom teacher. Don't complain about a problem without offering a solution. ❞

With a solution in mind I approached my public school's Home and School Association (HSA) about the terribly antiquated, rusted old water fountains students were reluctant to use. The fancy new filtered water filling stations seen in modern facilities cost less than $1,000. Surely one or two could be worked into the discretionary budget?

Turns out I was far from the first to inquire. All that was required was a bit of a push. And through the teamwork of the HSA, the principal, another invested teacher, and myself, two brand-new water fountains were installed within months of the original discussion. It proved that the red tape isn't always as thick as we imagine—sometimes you can cut it with a pair of safety scissors.

Apart from change that affects the whole school or classroom, the biggest thing parents can do is to pack their own healthy lunches and snacks to circumvent the unhealthy school lunches found in most areas.

Philadelphia public schools now offer free school lunches, regardless of your economic status. It is a blessing for children whose parents can't afford to provide adequate nutrition. But the quality of the prepackaged, reheated school lunches is notorious. In fact, less than one-third of schools even have full-service kitchens capable of preparing foods on site.

In July 2014, when the School District of Philadelphia's food service provider was up for new contract bids, students campaigned against the decade-long mainstay provider of frozen, pre-plated lunches. Revolution Foods, an innovative company providing healthy, fresh meals to schools, was one of two contract competitors. Despite pushback from students and parents, the notoriously litigious incumbent won the contract again.

I shudder from the sight of the Styrofoam trays and the knowledge that, on many days, chocolate milk is literally the only beverage served.

I am fortunate to be able to afford to pack my children healthy lunches. That doesn't mean they won't be trading their carrot sticks for Tastykakes—I can only beg for mercy. Some schools allow students to place their leftovers on a communal table for others to pick from. While it sounds like a good way to reduce food waste, it also offers the opportunity for children to make poor choices. And it's of particular concern for moms like Gina whose child has food sensitivities.

66 *Our child was given Skittles as a reward for hitting her goals with the occupational therapist. This had been after we'd removed artificial dyes and flavors from her diet and saw a marked improvement in social skills and behaviors. This is one time that I've felt fortunate to have an Individualized Education Program (IEP)—we made a provision that she was not allowed to have any food not provided by her parents. Additionally,*

my kids have food sensitivities, so the list of no-nos in their diet is long. Our school and community is often based around food events, so there have been years where avoiding snacks has been a challenge with teachers who believe frequent snacking is good. It's something I need to personally manage frequently, like being in the classroom on event days, especially when we are trying out elimination diets. **"**

But parents can't always be this hands-on, particularly when their children are older and require independence. When Janelle's daughter started 7th grade, she was quickly greeted with junk food galore.

" *Within the first week, they had a morning celebration and parents were encouraged to contribute food and drinks. My daughter told me people were bringing donuts, cupcakes, and soda, and I groaned. Why do they think this is a good way to start a child's day? Ironically, it's the physical education teacher hosting this celebration. Worse yet, these celebrations are supposed to happen two to four times per month depending on how many birthdays there are. It makes me sick. We're mindful at home about artificial colors and eating organic, but I know my kids will have these things at friends' houses and elsewhere. I don't sweat that. But to have a PE educator feed a classroom of kids a pile of sugar-laden junk food for breakfast blows my mind. If we aren't on the same page about basic nutrition, how will we ever see eye-to-eye about indoor air quality and toxic cleaning products and everything else that compromises our kids' health?* **"**

Lori Popkewitz Alper, who blogs at groovygreenlivin.com, says it's always amazed her that her children's school lunches include either milk or juice as a side, but water isn't an option.

" *At one point my kids mentioned they could purchase water for an additional 50 cents. With obesity issues looming for many American children, providing either a caloric juice or chocolate milk selection doesn't seem like a reasonable lunch option.* **"**

Bettina Elias Siegel is a nationally recognized commentator on issues relating to children and food policy who blogs at thelunchtray .com. In 2012, Bettina launched a petition that garnered more than 250,000 signatures and led the USDA to change its policy on "lean, finely textured beef" (aka "pink slime") in school food ground beef. In 2014, she scored another victory with a petition targeting the use of chicken processed in China in school meals.

Bettina first became involved in school food reform in 2010 when she joined a parent committee formed to advise the district on its school menus. Back then, the district was requiring children to take a packet of animal crackers every day at breakfast, which she was told would provide needed iron from fortified white flour. She was so dismayed by serving cookies at breakfast that she became interested in learning more about how the National School Lunch Program works and wanted to share that newfound knowledge with other parents.

Bettina concurs that improving the lunches in public school is a much tougher proposition than doing so in private schools.

66 *The federal government heavily regulates public school meals and also provides the funding for them. So, at the district level, the only real choice is the menu itself, which must conform with federal nutrition requirements and be purchased on a very limited budget. At the individual school level, there's often almost no input regarding what appears on lunch trays.* **99**

But Bettina says the good news is that with the Healthy, Hunger-Free Schools Act of 2010, we saw sweeping improvements to the nutritional standards for public school meals, including more whole grains, fruits, and vegetables, and less sodium.

In fact, the meals served in public schools are nutritionally balanced and do a decent job of nourishing the millions of kids who rely on them every day. But due to financial constraints, districts are often forced use highly processed food. For parents who would prefer to avoid that, their best bet is packing a lunch from home.

Bettina says while it can be hard to change school meals, parents can contact their district to discuss healthier school food options, keeping in mind that districts have about $1 per child per meal to spend on food.

66 *Putting aside the issue of school meals, parents can also do a lot to change the food culture at a school. Parents can raise funds for a salad bar (provided the district agrees to stock it with food), ask the district to no longer provide flavored milk at lunch, or set policies to help curb or eliminate junk food fundraising or the presence of junk food in classrooms.* 99

When I was in school, half the students had boxes of M&Ms and Starbursts strapped to them, selling candy as an effort to raise money for the marching band or Key Club. As a parent entering a cash-strapped public school I fully expected to be bombarded with catalogs for scented candles and cookie dough. I was ready to be annoyed, and I was ready to fight.

My jaw dropped when, on the third day of school, my son came home with a catalog for Equal Exchange, a provider of organic and fair trade coffee and chocolate. The note read, *"Thanks to Ms. Greenberg and her 8th grade class who petitioned the PTA to offer items that were fair trade. Their service learning project with a community nonprofit centered around learning about child labor."*

I didn't have to do a thing because the kids already did it for themselves.

As parents, it's difficult to give up control to schools. We may question testing methods, teaching styles, curriculum, or communication. And it's hard to know when to be an advocate and when to take a backseat. But parents and schools across the country have proven that we can create healthier environments for our children. Sometimes it takes a federal mandate, sometimes it takes a strong PTA, and sometimes, more often than you may think, all you need to do is ask.

T I P S for Improving Schools

☑ If teacher asks for hand sanitizer or sanitizing wipes on the school supply list, purchase disinfectants that use safer active ingredients and no synthetic fragrance, like EO Products, CleanWell, or Seventh Generation Wipes. If you can afford to, offer to purchase a case for the whole classroom or see if other parents are willing to chip in with you.

☑ Find other parents who share your values and will back you up. There's strength in numbers.

☑ Start small, with one particular item you'd like to see changed or improved. If you can find a way to show the financial difference would be negligible or even beneficial, you have your best ammunition.

☑ Explore avenues for outside funding for school eco-initiatives. Green Apple Program by The Center for Green Schools at the US Green Building Council (USGBC) gives individuals, companies, and organizations the opportunity to help transform schools into healthier spaces. The year 2015 yielded 617 projects across the globe, from educational events to clean up, planting, gardening, and e-waste recycling drives. Additional funding is available from Recyclebank's Green Schools Program, where Recyclebank members can donate points to fund school greening projects across the country.

CHAPTER 10

Can I Afford to Be This Conscious?

Making the Most of Every Green Dollar

COMING OF AGE in the generation somewhere between X and Y, I've noticed a particular dissonance with the older generations when it comes to economic independence.

It seems that for much of the mid-20th century, the average middle-class family survived quite easily on one income. Whether the breadwinner—almost always the male—was a construction worker or an insurance salesman, he could generally support a suburban home, two cars, two college educations, and a golden retriever.

Somewhere between Winona Ryder's '90s generation racking up the phone bill calling psychic friends in *Reality Bites* and the current boom of millennials upgrading their iPhones and updating their Instagrams, things got a lot more complicated.

We aren't just putting three square meals on the table and settling for TV dinners. Organic whole wheat bread costs some extra dough. Add that to the locally handmade toys, Suzuki music lessons, Montessori schools, unlimited data plans, and hybrid SUVs, and you really need to be bringing home the free-range, grass-fed bacon to survive.

Clearly, times are hard enough without the added expense of socially and environmentally conscious goods, which can bulk up the price tag.

Zoe Alexander, TV personality and author, says she is alarmed by how much more earth-friendly products can cost. But she feels it is a small price to pay for peace of mind.

66 *Instead of $5 for a big jar of baby wash at the supermarket, I pay $11.99 for a small bottle of the natural, organic stuff. But you start to think, over the course of a lifetime, if you can prevent something like cancer, then you're still ahead of the curve even though you're spending more money.* 99

New mom Felicia says she will forego her personal needs to spend more on organic food for her daughter.

66 *I just want the very best for Isabella, so I buy her all healthy and organic food, and if the bill is a little high, so be it. She's worth every cent. I just don't spend a lot of money on myself anymore. I don't get my nails or hair done as often as I used to—or it seems at all anymore.* 99

There's a reason organic has gotten a bad rep as "pretentious." Shopping organic is almost always more expensive. Whether it's food or clothing, various factors lead to higher overheads for organic cotton and berries.

Dr. Corinne Alexander, agricultural economics professor at Purdue University, says producing organic crops requires significantly more labor and results in lower yields. But while traditional laborious farm practices will probably never be able to compete with the simplicity of chemical spraying, prices could come down somewhat as the supply creeps closer to the demand.

66 *The supply within the US does not even come close to meeting the demand, and a lot of the organic products being sold here are imported. Because we don't have that critical mass of supply, it adds all of the additional transportation and logistics costs of getting it to the grocery store.* 99

The European union actually pays organic growers through subsidies, but that practice is unlikely to come to the US anytime soon.

The good news is that as demand rises, prices have already begun to come down. Because we are voting with our dollars, you can buy a reasonably priced pound of grass-fed meat at Costco and organic coconut oil at Walmart. I've seen organic avocados priced down next to conventional in the supermarket. There's still a socioeconomic discrepancy, but it doesn't seem completely insurmountable with a careful eye, a stack of coupons, and a membership to your local discount warehouse.

There are even a few forward-thinking programs to ease the socioeconomic burden, such as some farmers' markets accepting or even doubling the value of stamps from food assistance plans like WIC, SNAP, and Medicaid.

Marissa says green living isn't found on the $1 clearance rack, but it doesn't have to be expensive.

66 *I find a lot of my greener cleaning products in Target, and they aren't much more than the conventional brands. I even find some of my organic food items at the Aldi discounted supermarket chain.* 99

Lynn, a grandmother and green living author in Renton, WA, says she thinks "going crazy" trying to afford to live green and buy organic is a function of our cultural bias toward wanting and believing everything should be easy for us. She points to the fact that food is relatively cheap in the US. We pay less for it as a percentage of income than the vast majority of countries in the world. According to the Economic Research Service (ERS), a branch of the United States Department of Agriculture, Americans spend about 10 percent of their incomes on food in the home. In less developed countries, such as India and the Philippines, at-home food expenditures often account for more than 50 percent of a household's budget.[1]

And it's not just compared to other countries that the difference is profound. Between 1960 and 2013, disposable income spent on all food fell from 17.5 to 9.9 percent on average.[2] This drop occurred because prices of other consumer goods outpaced the price of food, and incomes rose at a faster rate than food prices.[3] But, as documented by films like *The Story of Stuff*, cheap things often have serious hidden costs, like unfair labor practices, factory farming, genetically engineered livestock, and wasteful manufacturing.

Lynn notes that another result of cheap food is a shift in our priorities.

66 *We take food for granted. We put having cable, cell phones, and cars ahead of food. We expect it to be cheap. So when we have to pay more, we get upset and say things like, 'It's too expensive.' In reality, this whole issue comes down to choice. Where do we want to spend our money? Once we understand the reasons why we ought to consider buying from greener companies and buying organic and make peace with that, it becomes a lot easier to say, 'Yes, it may cost more, but it's worth it.'* **99**

Ryan, a father of two in Philadelphia, says that until recently, he and his wife considered themselves eco- and health-conscious "as it was convenient and affordable for them."

66 *When you see a brand that's much cheaper than the organic you think, 'Oh, what's really the difference?'* **99**

But a recent realization, due in part to frustration over his daughter's severe peanut allergy, has him taking a second look at the difference in ingredients and being willing to spend a little more for the organic brands.

66 *If getting these things out of our lives is going to make us healthy and live longer, then paying a few extra bucks is well worth it.* **99**

But the crux of sustainability is consuming less. If you are doing it right, greener living should save you money—or at least enough money to compensate for the price of organic grapes.

As the years go on, Americans are collecting more items and taking up more actual space. The average size of a new American home in 1950 was 983 square feet; by 2014, it was 2,600 square feet—with fewer people living there, to boot.[4] This means the average person takes up more than three times the space we did 65 years ago.

Add to that our country's $22 billion personal storage industry, and we are working extremely hard to both collect things, and then store them.

We've been trained to think that buying less and avoiding the consumption of needless stuff is almost un-American. But studies have shown that, in the long run, experiences make people happier than possessions. And there is plenty to back up the notion that a clutter-free life feels more spiritually abundant, accounting for the popularity of movements like the Buy Nothing Project—a Facebook-based project centered on goodwill and a sharing economy—and books like Marie Kundo's *The Life Changing Magic of Tidying Up*.

Leslie Garrett, author of *The Virtuous Consumer*, also maintains that true green living will inevitably save money.

❝ *I think so many people think that living green means buying as much as ever, just buying the 'eco-friendly' version. But our consumption levels have to decrease if we really want to create change. I often say, sometimes the greenest product is the one we don't buy.* ❞

Leslie believes changes like making your own cleaning supplies, washing clothing in cold water, regulating your thermostat, and buying secondhand will save more than enough money to compensate for buying organic necessities.

Jen Boynton, editor of triplepundit.com, says she doesn't buy green per se, but she shops mindfully.

❝ *I consider durability, effectiveness, need, ethical sourcing, and environmental impact with all my purchases. I don't think it's more expensive, especially since the process always includes figuring out whether I actually need the product at all. Not buying anything is always the cheapest and greenest option.* ❞

Betsy Escandon, who blogs at eco-novice.com, says she discovered that green changes and choices come in a variety of shapes and sizes and have a way of balancing each other out.

" Certain green choices are expensive, like buying an all-natural bed free of flame-retardant chemicals. But many green choices, like making your own food, household cleaners, or even personal products, will save you money while keeping toxic or unknown ingredients out of your family's bodies. "

Additionally, Betsy says, shifting from disposables to reusables, such as rechargeable batteries or cloth diapers, might require an initial small investment but will pay you back many times over in the long term. And choosing to purchase quality durable goods and repairing what you already own instead of buying the cheapest and newest version available is doubly beneficial.

" I have found it helpful, and often necessary budget-wise, to pair expensive changes with money-saving ones. For example, instead of spending thousands of dollars on disposable diapers for your baby, use cloth diapers and spend that money on buying a nontoxic bed for baby instead. In my own household, by making most meals as well as bread and snacks from scratch while purchasing fewer packaged and convenience foods, we have been able to afford to purchase mostly organic products. "

Inevitably, we are still going to cringe at the price of organic cotton and grass-fed beef. But at its deepest root, green living curbs excessive spending, putting formerly squandered money back in the pockets of a wiser consumer.

The height of the economic crisis coined the term *recessionista*, a shopper who maintained style with savvy and a renewed sense of purchase discernment. The new consumer embraces old-fashioned practicality and creative resourcefulness paired with the ease of coupon clicking from her laptop.

There are hundreds of ways to save money while greening your lifestyle. And the new sharing economy has made it that much more accessible. Before buying anything new, I check my neighborhood Buy Nothing Group, as well as Yerdle, where everything is entirely free, save for shipping. If I just want a great secondhand bargain, I go to Poshmark for women's clothing and Craigslist or eBay for anything else.

When I really need to buy something new, I try to support triple bottom-line businesses that care about the planet, people, and profit. B Corporation status is one good way to find these companies, or you can shop at trusted retailers (outlined in Chapter 13). And you can still save a lot by being a savvy shopper. I am a big coupon connoisseur, and there are wonderful websites that offer great deals on green products and services:

- Coupon sites for natural and organic products include mambo sprouts.com, thegreenbacksgal.com, and organicdeals.com.
- Whole Foods has launched a new rewards program complete with in-app coupons.
- Berry Cart: app with cash back on select natural brands.
- No matter what you're shopping for online, always visit ebates. com first to get up to 15 percent back on your purchases. This no-strings-attached site has earned me close to $2,000 in cash back over the past ten years. Also, don't forget to do an online search for coupon codes.

Just try to keep in mind that not every "green gadget" on the market is an eco-savvy purchase. There's a fine line between supporting the green economy and simply buying more stuff.

Shel Horowitz, a green business profitability expert and author of *Guerrilla Marketing to Heal the World*, says it can be counterintuitive to sustainability to always purchase the most eco-friendly new thing.

66 *If you're buying a new furnace because your old one is down to 70 percent efficient and you're basically pumping hydrocarbons into the air, then a $5,000 furnace can be a very green purchase. On the other hand, if you buy a pair of eco-friendly sneakers when you already have a pair of perfectly good sneakers, I'd say wait until your sneakers have a few holes in them.* 99

So if you're thinking about trading in your gas-guzzling SUV for a hybrid, your best option is to see if it's possible to drive less altogether. But if you have an inevitable 100-mile daily commute on your hands, the gas savings may be reason to accelerate that purchase.

Diane MacEachern, author of *Big Green Purse*, is an expert in making greener purchases that will save consumers money in the long run. She says you can actually save thousands of dollars a year by choosing the most sustainable product or service available. And when you do, it creates a powerful incentive for conventional companies to clean up their act.

66 *A 99 cent sponge lasts as long as 24 rolls of paper towels, which costs $53.99 at Costco. In other cases, there are trade-offs. Many people won't buy organic milk because it costs a dollar more per gallon. But some of those same people may spend $10 or $15 a week on bottled water, which has no health benefits and takes a terrible toll on the planet. Exchange the bottled water for organic milk, and maybe a one-time purchase of a water filter for big savings over time.* 99

Diane says that when making a purchase, she looks for tangible differences in water and energy use, her personal health, and waste.

66 *For example, I finally replaced my big old television with a sleek, thin, lightweight LED model. The new TV uses far less energy than the old one, and because I can plug in a Roku to stream programs, I was able to get rid of cable. In addition to saving about $75 a month on my cable bill, I'm also saving energy because cable boxes are such energy hogs. That decision made perfect sense.* 99

Her mantra is first buy less; then buy the greenest option available to meet your needs. And think long term.

66 *Compared to a regular incandescent, an LED light bulb will cost a couple dollars more in the short term. But that same incandescent would cost you about $160 more to operate over its lifetime.* 99

Overall, if we are more mindful with our purchasing—reducing, reusing, and repurposing along the way—we can ultimately save substantial dollars to vote with. And every time we vote with our dollars—buying or even not buying something—we send a message to improve the accessibility and affordability of a growing green economy.

Money-Saving Ideas from Green Bloggers

❝ *One of the things we did in order to make buying personal care products, cleaning supplies, and organic dry goods more affordable was organize a co-op through Frontier Natural Products Co-op. It cost about $20 to set the whole thing up, and I spend maybe an hour each month coordinating with a group of moms in my area to place a large group order. This gets us wholesale pricing on items like shampoo, deodorant, bulk spices, tea, and lots more. We end up paying about 50 percent of what we would have paid in a grocery store for these same items.* ❞

—Carissa Bonham, creativegreenliving.com

❝ *I try to buy in bulk at Costco to decrease the cost or wait until items are on sale at the grocery store. Eating in season also helps with prices. And, of course, growing what you can at home.* ❞

—Anna Hackman, green-talk.com

❝ *You can save money by buying in bulk and freezing. Things to freeze include organic fruits, organic vegetables, grass-fed meat, large batches of soup and baked goods like muffins, pancakes, waffles, smoothies, and bulk cooked beans (cheaper and safer than buying canned). You can also buy frozen organic produce more cheaply than fresh.* ❞

—Jenny Bradford, living-consciously.com

❝ *Buy one thing that can serve many purposes. For example, certified organic coconut oil can be used for cooking, skin hydration, makeup removal, and so much more! If you break the cost down by the number of times you use it, it actually becomes very affordable.* ❞

—Rachel Sarnoff, mommygreenest.com

Make Money, Do Social Good, and Avoid Landfills:
How to Do the Most Good Discarding Unwanted Items

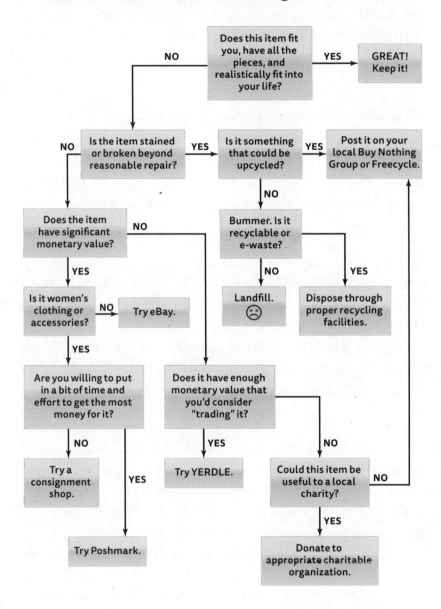

Do More with Less: A Few Easy Bare(ly) Homesteading Recipes to Help You Preserve in a Pinch

Pickling 101

Want to make the most of a bumper crop of cucumbers, string beans, or carrots? Here's how to pickle—no canning necessary. Boil one cup of white vinegar with one cup of water. Add a few pinches of some basic pickling spices like dill, bay leaves, garlic, mustard seed, salt, and sugar. You can even spice it up with peppers and chilies. Pour the simmering liquid into a jar with the veggies sliced anyway you prefer, stick in the fridge for a couple hours, and voila!

Pump up the Jam

Plenty of fruit? Here's how to make jam. Cut up fruit and stir in a saucepan over medium heat along with the juice of one lemon. Frequently stir that bubbling pot. After about 15 minutes, add in a bit of sugar—you really don't need very much with a sweet fruit. Keep stirring over heat. It will miraculously become jam-like and you will know it when you see it. This shouldn't take more than another five to ten minutes. You don't want to cook it too long or the sugar will caramelize and make everything taste funky. Take off heat, put in a jar, and let cool. Keep in the fridge as long as you'd keep ordinary opened jam.

Stock Up

It's cheaper to buy a whole organic chicken than to buy it in parts—but you have no use for that meatless back portion and the dinky little wings! Thirty-two ounces of organic chicken stock costs about $5. This recipe yields roughly four quarts and costs nothing. In your largest pot, throw whatever raw chicken parts you won't be using (as well as cooked bones) and fill about three-quarters up with water. You definitely want to toss some salt, pepper, and at least half an onion in there, but with everything else, you can get creative with whatever is around the house—carrots, celery, garlic, bay leaves, parsley, rosemary, and thyme. Bring to a boil and then simmer with a lid for three or four hours. Drain out the solid bits and freeze the rest in portions.

Don't Leave a Crumb

Leftover bread? Breadcrumbs or croutons become easy saves. Break up the bread into easily toastable chunks. Drizzle with some garlic and olive oil and cook at 350 degrees for about 15 minutes or until it is crispy but not burned. Now you have croutons. For crumbs, throw in a bag with some dried herbs (oregano works nicely) and beat the hell out of it with the back of a pan. This is therapeutic.

CHAPTER 11

Aw, You Shouldn't Have. No, Really, You Shouldn't Have

When Family and Friends Won't Support Your Green Habit

YOU'VE LOADED UP the crib with wooden toys, mastered the art of five-minute organic baby food, and have recycling down to a science. And then Grandma comes to visit.

For all their well-meaning wishes and abundance of love for their grandchildren, many of our parents come from the generation where formula was queen and Pine-Sol was king. They were raised to throw cigarettes out windows and leave their Raisinets wrappers on the movie theater floor.

Some boomer parents see my generation as undue worriers who exaggerate the problems. And I'm not the only one fighting an uphill battle for the greater good of the next generation. Honi says her extended family has created a "forever challenge" for her.

❝ *It's OK that they don't get it, but I feel like they also don't respect it. They live to 'spoil' our children with junk and candy. We've tried to have them understand that they can spoil our children with love and time and traditions. Teach our children how to bake your favorite cookies or how to work in your garden. That is making memories. My friends and I set up a text chain when we visit our parents and in-laws so we can vent about the flowing unhealthy food options, the useless toys, and railroading of parents.* 99

Rebecca says her parents believe she's manufacturing these concerns.

66 *They think I'm largely imagining this stuff—that it's a sign of being unfulfilled and overly self-involved or something. They've never said this directly, but they make sarcastic comments about things like the cage-free organic eggs and the fact that I refuse to use fabric softener sheets and have all-natural latex mattresses.* 99

Rebecca says going to her in-laws causes her to walk a fine line between complete and utter disregard for the environment and overstepping her bounds and tending to their nonexistent recycling.

66 *They have a closet chock-full of highly toxic chemical cleansers, air fresheners, cheap ultra-smelly candles, and extra-strength fabric softener sheets. Plus, they only drink bottled water and don't recycle anything. I really try to accommodate, but sometimes I can't, and I rummage the trash and pick out 15 little water bottles and endless stacks of recyclable mail.* 99

Amy Wilson, actress and author of *When Did I Get Like This?*, feels frustrated that her in-laws still use Saran Wrap on her kids' microwaved leftovers when she's not looking.

66 *I think there's more of a sense of futility about it all in the baby boomer generation. I try to motivate them by telling them it's about protecting their grandchildren's planet.* 99

Rachel Sarnoff, former CEO of Healthy Child Healthy World and blogger at mommygreenest.com, says every Halloween she aims to be a good example for trick-or-treaters, armed with fair-trade organic chocolate minis.

❝ *My kids complain that I'm going to be the crazy lady on the corner giving out crappy candy. But then, without fail, the day before the holiday my mother-in-law drops off her contribution to our annual party: a giant bowl full of what I consider truly the worst candy. But what can I do? She's my mother-in-law. I grit my teeth and give it out, hoping that it runs out fast so we can break out the good stuff.* **❞**

Dani Klein, comedian and author of *Afterbirth: Stories You Won't Read in a Parenting Magazine*, says she had a huge fight with her mother the first year of her son's life.

❝ *She simply could not wait to give them ice cream, and my mother has a real problem with boundaries, as do most people who tell you how you should be eating. I try to get to the bad stuff before the boys even see it, but if they do, I explain that it's not going to make them feel good and usually let them choose one item and throw the rest away. That goes for plastic junk, too. I can't stand it. It's such a waste. I sound so cranky. That's me, cranky mom.* **❞**

We, the new generation of frustrated mothers, have tried gently explaining our concerns to our families and even register holiday wish lists with appropriate products. But our parents simply couldn't resist buying our little munchkins those Teenage Mutant Ninja Turtles pencil cases (laced with cadmium and phthalates, according to a 2013 report by healthytoys.org, an environmental advocacy organization).[1]

Jennifer Grayson, environmental journalist, eco-etiquette expert, and mother of two, says family members routinely unload cheap toys on her children.

❝ *We just keep repeating the message that the girls don't have room for many toys and when people come to visit to please just bring themselves. And when it's birthday time or holiday time and family members ask what the kids would like, we suggest 'experience' gifts like art classes or tickets to a show, or if there's one 'thing' that the girls really* *want, a well-made version that will last for years to come. It's taken a few years, but most of our friends and family 'get it' now, though it's not always possible to preempt everything.* **99**

In the meantime, we know Grandma's going to wonder where's Johnny's new toy truck, but we don't want the answer to be, "gradually leaching cadmium into his mouth." So what are we supposed to do with all this unwanted stuff?

Many of us simply pack up unwelcome offerings, re-gift them to less environmentally conscious friends, or give them to charities that will be happy to take anything. But is it in good conscience to give to someone who may not look a re-gifted non-wooden horse in its lead-painted mouth? By donating bags of plastic toys to shelters, we may be inadvertently poisoning less economically fortunate children.

Comedian and mother Lisa Landry says that when her mother sends her foreign-made, lead-painted toys—no matter how many times she asks her not to—she throws them out, believing they'll do less harm in a landfill than in a children's shelter.

66 *They have enough problems. They don't need slow toy-induced brain damage too.* **99**

Alas, the mountain of stuff grows, and while we know we should feel thankful for the abundance laid out before us, we also know we're better off without the contaminated clutter.

Chrissy is a firm believer in returning items to the big box stores from whence they came.

66 *I exchange gifts that don't fit in with our lifestyle. I've even gone as far as repackaging a recent birthday gift because it was ripped open by an enthusiastic gift-giver during the party. As soon as the guests left, I repackaged it and it's going back. It's like 30 plastic pieces which she already owned in wood.* **99**

Mom Melinda says that, while she would not re-gift an item she wouldn't want her own child to have, she would give it to a resale shop.

> ❝ I think giving something as a present is different than supplying a product for a store to sell as inventory where they likely have many of the same anyway. People looking for a product like that would probably buy it new anyway, and if they see it at a resale store for less, maybe they would buy it secondhand. ❞

Of course, Melinda says, anything that is clearly toxic—containing lead or the subject of a recall—only goes back to the original store or into the trash.

Jennifer Grayson has her own solutions for unwanted candy.

> ❝ If you really don't want to throw it away or let your kid eat it, you can always save it for piñata filler or even throw it in your emergency survival kit. Maybe you'll be happy to have that bag of gummy worms when the world is coming to an end. ❞

Swapping out the bad stuff is simple when your child is too young to notice. And then they discover the world, resplendent in Skittles and squirt guns. Scratch-and-sniff stickers at the doctor's office and the dreaded claw machine at Bounce U.

For a family with children older than age two, a typical three-day span is peppered with gummy bears from the dollar store, blue lollipops, and Munchkins, Munchkins everywhere.

Here's an excerpt from my life:

Day One—Preschool

7 AM: We make the children organic frozen waffles or the Cascadian Farm's organic version of Life cereal.

8:30 AM: They complain they're still hungry, so they eat Earth's Best fruit bars on the walk to school.

10 AM: Snack time at school. Sometimes it's fruit and sometimes it's ordinary supermarket snacks. And then there's pretzel day, when they eat massive soft pretzels, leading to:

12 PM: Lunch. Mostly uneaten, as seen by the remnants of organic peanut butter and jelly, fruit, and random leftovers.

3 PM: Afternoon snack at school. It's someone's birthday because it is always someone's birthday. And it's always Munchkins.

4 PM: At pick-up, I notice their hair smells like cheap shaving cream, requisite for preschool "water play" fun.

4:05 PM: We head to the park. I've brought some fruit and organic snack foods, but Johnny's parents have come armed with lollipops and Jane's parents have gummy worms in tow. My children no longer like what I have and beg to share their friends' snacks. Sometimes I say yes, sometimes I say no.

4:30 PM: The Mister Softee truck rolls up to the playground blaring its siren song. All the children run to the fence. Some of the kids get ice cream. Mine don't.

4:45 PM: A person dressed like the Nesquik bunny enters the park with an igloo full of "chocolate drink." We rapidly head out.

5:30 PM: We prepare a healthy, mostly organic dinner. My two-year-old crumples down on the kitchen floor and cries because she wants Cheddar Bunnies for dinner. My five-year-old son subsists on about six different things (because we have failed). But we will make damn sure those six things are organic, so Annie's Mac and Cheese is served.

6 PM: I prepare homemade fruit and almond milk ice cream in the Vitamix, peppered with the requisite chocolate chips. Sam wants real ice cream instead. He finally gives in and eats what I've made. Five minutes later, he complains that he is hungry again and eats four pickles, a cheese stick, and an errant Girl Scout cookie bought out of guilt from a friend's daughter.

Day Two—Saturday

7 AM: Breakfast

10 AM: Sam needs a haircut, so he is plied with healthy-ish snacks to prepare him for the ten minutes of captivity. After the haircut, he is offered a small cup of peanut M&Ms by the well-meaning barber and we let him eat them.

12 PM: A begrudgingly eaten and picked-at lunch.

12:30 PM: My parents arrive with three plastic Ninja Turtles and a bag of chocolate chip muffins, literally dotted with granulated sugar. I have fought with them about this ad nauseum, but I cannot win because it "gives them pleasure" to ply my children with what I consider to be junk. The kids eat the muffins.

1 PM: My parents want to give them Oreos. I say no. We fight. The kids cry.

1:30 PM: They want to know if they can take the kids to the drugstore to pick out some candy. I say no. The kids cry.

1:45 PM: The Ninja Turtles no longer have legs.

2 PM: My father insists that the television be on at all times, blaring commercials for McDonald's, Gatorade, and Frosted Flakes.

4 PM: We head out for one of the daily neighborhood festivals that make city living so great. I know this is one of those occasions where we'll want to splurge on pizza and ice cream with no thought about ingredients, and so we do. But since Sam has already gobbled down M&Ms, a giant sugar-coated muffin, and possibly other things snuck by my parents, this ice cream cone has put him over the top, and he is high-strung and freaking out. Covered in rainbow sprinkles, Evelyn is chewing on her shoe.

6 PM: We all go home and eat cereal and grapes.

6:30 PM: Sam is hungry again.

Day Three—Sunday

7 AM: Breakfast

9 AM: Sam and I take the dog for a walk and the dog drags us into the dry cleaners where he knows he will get a bone. And Sam knows he will get a small Hershey bar.

10 AM: The first birthday party of the day. It is at one of the many establishments where you must consume their provided cuisine—cardboard pizza and Hi-C. I am forced to go with the flow.

12 PM: Cake with blue icing.

12:30 PM: The new requisite piñata, pre-filled with candy I can't even believe still exists, like Laffy Taffy.

12:45 PM: A goody bag consisting of cheap plastic trinkets, temporary tattoos, and something sticky and blue.

2 PM: Birthday party No. 2. Same thing, different bounce house.

5 PM: Dinner. Hahaha!!!

People love to say, "It's just one lollipop—it won't kill them." Rest assured, my children are not sweet or toy deprived. They aren't living in some candy-crushed world where they can only eat things they've grown with their bare hands. We're simply trying to do a little bit better because we know what's in this stuff.

We know how it affects our children in the short term, and we're terrified of how it will harm them years down the line. We would be remiss and frankly, ignorant, to just let all hell break loose in a blaze of red dye and pesticides.

Spend a day in the shoes of a parent forced to fight in the universal food wars, and you will know that every crumb counts.

No amount of preaching or protecting will change the fact that some people have no interest in taking on the burden of environmental awareness. And when it's the people closest to us, sometimes having our children spend time with them is an exercise in editing.

Mom Betsy says she does her best to shape her children's environment and explain their choices when they contrast with others'. But she also wants to make sure she doesn't sound too judgmental.

❝ *I remind them that they don't need to share their opinions about other people's food choices.* ❞

Rebecca finds solace in reminding herself that time in other people's domains won't entirely undermine the values instilled on her home turf.

❝ *My attitude is that when I'm in your house, I'm not going to say a word about the air freshener in the bathroom, triclosan in the soap, or* the flame retardants in the remote control the baby is gnawing on. I might make an exploratory comment, and if they seem interested, then I'm ready to hop up on my (vegetable-based) soapbox and enlighten them. If not, then I remember that we'll only be spending a little while in a less-than-ideally-healthy environment. **"**

Jennifer Grayson agrees that if a grandparent wants to take them out for ice cream or let them have a lollipop at the bank, it's not the end of the world.

" I have to believe from my own upbringing where I was allowed to eat real candy on Halloween and probably ate more than my fair share of blue icing birthday cake at parties, that if you feed kids real, wholesome food 95 percent of the time, they will grow up to be adults with a taste for real, wholesome food. **"**

David Alan Basche, star of TV Land's "The Exes" and father of a six-year-old, believes in letting the results of poor eating speak for themselves.

" After a while, the grandparents see with their own eyes what happens when their granddaughter has too little sleep, too much sugar, or not enough greens and quality protein. Dealing with a sluggish, irritable kid sleeping over will make you pay attention really fast to what you feed her. **"**

Sometimes we have to treat people a bit like we treat our children. It may take some handholding, but even then, you know what they say about leading a horse to filtered tap water. Unless you're paying for babysitting services—and want to spend your spare time reviewing a nanny cam—there is no absolute way to ensure your wishes will be upheld.

Unfortunately, it often takes diagnosis or disaster to be the catalyst for an individual's greater shift. One in three children has food allergies, asthma, ADHD, or autism. Cancer is the leading cause of death by disease in American children.[2,3]

Robyn O'Brien, a former food industry analyst, author of *The Unhealthy Truth*, and founder of the AllergyKids Foundation, believes foresight is a gift.

66 *As frustrating as it may seem, we have been given this privilege and gift of being able to see this early. If someone can't see it yet, you can't just hit them over the head. You have to just be grateful that you've been able to see this and be there for when they are ready to take the blinders off. You can't wear the blinders anymore when your child is diagnosed with diabetes or a food allergy.* 99

But some people simply aren't ready to confront an inconvenient reality.

66 *You have to be fiercely strong to be able to confront that former version of yourself and think, 'Oh my God, what did I do?'* 99

When faced with the choice of grinning and bearing it versus speaking up for our convictions, even the latter can often feel futile.

Syndi Seid, etiquette trainer and founder of San Francisco-based Advanced Etiquette, recommends that instead of accusing someone of doing something wrong, determine why the person seems reluctant to change his or her ways for the greater good of the environment.

66 *Times change, and new and better ways to handle things are learned every day. Recognize that old habits die hard. Work on finding an amicable resolution together, supported by the advantages and positive outcomes of the choices you will make.* 99

As a grandmother, Lynn Colwell understands that many grandparents think they know what's best. But Lynn, who wrote the book *Celebrate Green!* with her daughter Corey, believes that when parents use the right approach, most grandparents will come on board (however grudgingly).

66 *If your mother or mother-in-law is of a different opinion, acknowledging her expertise as a parent will go a long way toward helping her*

make the shift. Focus on your gratitude for providing a good upbringing for you or your mate. It might help if you ask if she had different ideas about raising kids than her mother did and if so, what was it like for her to counter those ideas. For example, breastfeeding was a big one for me. My mother thought that only women who could not afford to buy formula would do it. **"**

In addition to careful dialogue and gentle prodding, the experts emphasize reinforcing positive behavior. If that means giving your parents a biscuit every time they drop something in the recycling bin, so be it.

The best we can do for our children is to minimize exposure to the products and practices—and people—we don't feel comfortable with. A weekend stay with Grandpa will not likely turn your kid into a cigar-smoking, soda-chugging lush. And who knows, maybe your child's voice will be the impetus to finally get Grandma on board with garden composting.

T I P S for Dealing with Family and Friends

☑ Reward positive behavior. Tell others how clever and environmentally savvy they are.

☑ Make a point no one can argue with. People may dispute the relevance of your efforts and even try to fight science, but it's difficult to debate how you feel.

☑ Passing along things we wouldn't trust for our own health is a tricky topic, but throwing the contaminants into the trash cycle isn't doing much good either. Save up unwanted items and seek out the most return-friendly store or resale shop.

☑ If they don't sympathize, minimize. You don't have to ban people, places, or things—just keep exposure to a healthy minimum.

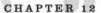

CHAPTER 12

Four Coach Seats and a Million White Cotton Towels

Can One Flight Undo All Your Green Good?

VACATIONS ARE A TIME TO RELAX—or relax as much as you possibly can with two children at Disney World.

In that respect, I'm guilty of easing my eco-consciousness a bit while away from home. I don't travel particularly often, and when I do, I try to carry a refillable water bottle and use the hotel towels more than one day. But I am also prone to letting go—not searching too hard for a recycling bin or buying a few bottles of water after passing airport security.

One of the worst culprits for ecological sin is air travel. One round-trip flight from New York to Europe or San Francisco creates a warming effect equivalent to two or three tons of carbon dioxide per person. The average American generates about 19 tons of carbon dioxide a year—probably significantly less if you walk, bike, or take public transit to work.[1]

In fact, if you don't drive much and live an eco-conscious lifestyle, flying could be by far the largest part of your carbon footprint.

I used to wrongly view airplanes as a type of "public transit," with my footprint not factoring in since the flights would take off with or without me. I also believed air travel may be decreasing, with the rise in virtual communication.

But in reality the volume of air travel has increased much faster than gains in flight-fuel efficiency. Recent reports say the demand for air travel will likely double by 2035.[2] Personally, I'd rather get a Pap smear than go through an airport security line, and flying coach rivals the New York subway at rush hour.

But humans are susceptible to wanderlust, and it's educational, eye-opening, and enjoyable to visit other places, countries, and cultures. Who doesn't have the pyramids of Egypt on their bucket list? (OK, I don't.)

But will our yearning for travel abroad tarnish the natural wonders of the world?

Mom Rosie says that, while she feels a strong responsibility toward her family, community, and planet, her life is nothing if not "an awkward compromise."

❝ Yes, we use cloth diapers, buy mostly organic produce, don't eat meat, and have disavowed nasty chemical products in our house. But my biggest source of guilt right now is the amount we travel. We've traveled by plane at least three weekends a month for the past several months. Not only am I exhausted, but I can also see my personal ozone hole following me around. ❞

For actress Alysia Reiner, travel is a necessary part of her business.

❝ This is my most guilty eco-truth considering I fly so much for work— and for pleasure, too. I can't Skype in a performance, but I can Skype into meetings or take the subway. As for pleasure, well, you can't Skype Bora Bora. ❞

With half of her husband's family in California while they live in Texas, Jenny's family makes several plane trips each year.

❝ For us, it is a function of travel time. We don't have an extra week to add to our time off to make driving a reasonable alternative, and trains and buses are not a great idea with very young children. ❞

New mom Jeanette says she thinks about her carbon emissions when flying, but she can't always take off the extra time to drive. So she compromises by packing light (weight = emissions) and driving for shorter trips.

66 *We do drive a good amount for vacation, since we have two dogs to haul around with us. For family vacations within 700 miles, we definitely drive. Our limit is ten hours in the car. We also buy most breakfasts and lunch food at a grocery store and bring containers so we don't buy single packaging goodies left and right. But we do splurge a little bit by going out to eat for dinners and getting coffee and ice cream.* 99

Jeanette recognizes the challenge of vacationing and showing our children new experiences and cultures while keeping personal carbon emissions in check.

66 *I think it's a trade-off, and we make as many sustainable choices as possible once we get there. We often camp or stay in a cabin or Airbnb at our destination to provide a more family-like experience, which to us means eating in and making green choices, like local market food shopping.* 99

Jen Boynton, editor of triplepundit.com, says sometimes nothing replaces an in-person meeting and conferences are a good way to get the most bang for your emissions.

66 *The benefit of conferences is that you can meet with many, many people at once, so it does reduce the number of necessary trips overall.* 99

Irene Lane, sustainable tourism consultant and founder of eco-travel site greenloons.com, explains that carbon offsets present an opportunity for people to counter their carbon emissions by investing in certain forestry, renewable energy, or development projects. Airlines such as KLM, Qantas, and United offer carbon offset programs that allow consumers to offset their flight at the point of sale.

But Lane recommends first checking the credentials for any carbon offsetting scheme by looking for independent certification (the Climate Action Reserve and Green-e are two recommended by the National Resource Defense Fund).

❝ If you want to determine your approximate carbon emissions, jot down your travels in the last year, locate your latest utility statements, and fill in the carbon calculator at carbonfootprint.com. ❞

Once we've arrived at our destinations, via plane, train, automobile, or cruise ship (another eco-sin I'm a sucker for), we must deal with accommodation and consumption choices while on holiday.

Unfortunately, the tourism industry is rife with greenwashing. In fact, New York environmentalist Jay Westerveld first coined the term greenwashing in 1986 after seeing a "Save Our Planet" towel use placard in a hotel bathroom. Towel reuse would purportedly help the hotel save water and to consequently "save the environment." However, Westerveld found that despite promises, these offending hotels put little effort toward waste reduction—and not washing as many linens saves the hotel money.

Lane says it should come as no surprise that many accommodations and touring companies have adopted terms such as "green" and "environmentally friendly" to attract customers.

❝ There are financially lucrative reasons for marketing hotels, restaurants, and vacation activities in this manner since surveys have indicated that travelers are willing to pay a premium for a product when they are aware that an organization is environmentally conscious. To be sure a hotel is truly sustainable, check that it has obtained an eco-certification that is recognized and/or approved by the Global Sustainable Tourism Council. ❞

Lane explains that true ecotourism focuses on the discovery of a natural or wildlife habitat in a manner that maximizes local economic and social goals while reducing the possibility of environmental degradation.

“ *It is through eco-certifications that travelers can be assured that the guiding company or eco-lodge supports local communities, emphasizes environmental education, sustains conservation efforts, efficiently utilizes scarce resources, minimizes tourist waste, and respects local cultural traditions.* ”

Even shopping at small family-run enterprises supports local business while avoiding tourist traps.

Mom Larisha says that when her family travels, they try to find local restaurants instead of chains, to support the local economy.

“ *Bonus points if they source locally and/or use organic. Otherwise, during vacations we use this time to ease up a bit on our other beliefs in order to create new experiences for our family.* ”

Mom Michelle travels to Malaysia once every three years to see family. It's a long flight, but she says her living experience is incredibly green simply by virtue of the culture and economy.

“ *We live nine in one condo with no dryer or dishwasher. Everything that needs to be dried gets hung up on one drying rack on the balcony.* ”

Michelle says she believes it's actually easier to be green when traveling because you are already living with less—one suitcase as opposed to a whole house.

“ *I think it's natural to want to stay out of malls and go to places you don't have at home. You're more inclined to want to experience what is unique and local as opposed to what is merely cheap and convenient. You're not focused on consuming, but experiencing.* ”

But apart from that major excursion, Michelle's family prefers to take advantage of all the culture easily accessible from her home in the Boston suburbs.

“ *I guess we are lucky living in the Northeast, because there is so much to see and do within driving distance. We do a lot of day trips but also keep an eye on what is happening locally. There is so much to experience close to home. I feel very fortunate in where I live. There aren't many places in this world where you can pull the car over and witness a Revolutionary War battle reenactment on your way to the grocery store.* 99

Betsy avoids travel as much as possible and has mastered the art of the "staycation," but her reasons are not about being eco-virtuous or even to save money.

66 *It's because I hate traveling with children. But instead of feeling pathetic or guilty about it, I can instead pat myself on the back and think about how I'm helping out my friend the planet.* 99

Staycations can vary from simply unplugging from devices for a few days, to checking out the local tourist attractions you've never bothered to see, to exploring local adventures like hiking, biking, sailing, or surfing.

Lane notes that there are many cultures, including Navajo, Ojibwe, Amish, and Creole, along with historical sites that children can immerse themselves in right here in the United States. In fact, many of these sites are discussed at length during social studies class—a helpful note for getting an approved school absence.

66 *As for longer-range trips, this is a personal decision each family must make for themselves. Luckily, we live in a world where technology helps to educate people about other far-reaching cultures. However, in my opinion, to be a globally responsible citizen is to experience a region, a people, a culture for oneself rather than through the filtered lens of another person's viewpoint or agenda.* 99

As much as I yearn to see the Seven Wonders of the World (or at least three or four of them), it's the extra baggage of whining, jet-lagged children that keeps me pretty much grounded. Carsickness dictates short road trips, and New Jersey is pretty much the closest thing we get to interstate travel.

Until my children are old enough to carry their own luggage, travel is relegated to an annual pilgrimage to Florida to see my parents and a society-mandated solitary trip to Disney World.

Fortunately, we live in a major cultural and historical hub. There's great hiking and natural reserves only 20 minutes away and a beach you can get to in the duration of one "Sesame Street" episode. Life is a staycation I'm happy to take.

Personally, I'm waiting for retirement for my next globetrotting adventures—a low-maintenance old woman with a backpack. The only diapers I will carry will be my own.

T I P S for Greener Travel

☑ Consider a "staycation" or a trip that avoids the need for flights. If you do fly, aim for a single longer trip versus multiple short vacations. Consider carbon offsets through reputable sites like terrapass.com or carbonfund.org.

☑ Don't pay for bottled water: if you're in an area with safe tap water, just use one bottle and refill. If at a hotel or on a cruise ship, visit the fitness center or spa for water fountains and coolers—maybe there will even be some cucumbers in them!

☑ BYO breakfast and snack food. If you don't have room in your suitcase, order Amazon or a local grocery service to the hotel for a stock of healthy snacks you don't have to pay hotel gift-shop prices for.

☑ Treat your hotel room like it's your own house by turning off the lights and air conditioning when you leave.

☑ Use public transportation, bike, or walk instead of opting for a car rental.

☑ Support the community you're visiting by purchasing food and other goods from local suppliers.

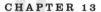

CHAPTER 13

Made With Real Ingredients

When Greenwashing Has You Completely Soaked

DESPITE ALL THE WONDERFUL eco-minded progress being made by existing and new companies, one thing remains disheartening: the amount of greenwashing—companies disingenuously spinning their products and policies as environmentally friendly.

Made with natural ingredients? So are cigarettes. So is cocaine. Name one thing on earth that does not contain some percentage of a natural ingredient—and remember water is a natural ingredient.

This kind of labeling has been proliferating on products for the past few years, as companies try to upgrade their green marketing way faster than they actually upgrade their manufacturing.

Have you ever seen something labeled "Made with Real Ingredients"? You know, versus imaginary ones.

A few years ago I opened the newspaper to find Procter & Gamble's "Future Friendly Brandsaver" which included slogans like "Save Energy with Tide Coldwater," "Sustainably Manufactured Charmin Mega Roll," and "Save Water with Cascade."

OK, so we're supposed to be happy that they use somewhat less energy in their plant that creates paper products from 100-percent virgin trees? You want us to feel good about using a dishwasher formula with sodium hypochlorite to avoid the pre-rinse? And all of this is touted as "creating a better future for our children," in advertisements with children skipping along with reusable bags filled with the company's products.[1,2]

Lately, companies seem to just look for the "greenest" thing about their brands to exploit for marketing purposes. Really not so different from saying, "We haven't shot a kitten in 30 years" or "We serve carrots in the break room."

Kleenex wants you to believe that only a single-use paper towel can truly dry your hands. Lysol coined the term "healthing" for spraying several of the Environmental Working Group's red-flag ingredients all over your house. Popular shampoo brands pack undefined fragrance and possible neurotoxic ingredients in plant-derived packaging and give it a nature-inspired name.[3,4]

Adryenn Ashley, producer, actress, and author of *Every Single Girl's Guide to Her Future Husband's Last Divorce*, realizes that the word "natural" has no definitive meaning.

 ❝ *Sometimes 'natural vanilla' really means beaver butt juice. Totally not kidding, look it up. And then, sometimes you think you're buying a small local brand only to find out it was bought by a big corporation who added some secret ingredients to make it more addictive.* **❞**

Companies grasp at straws to pull our green heartstrings. And, if we're not careful, it will work.

Carissa sent her eco-savvy husband out in search of nontoxic carpet shampoo, but was not thrilled with what he brought home.

 ❝ *He bought one that had some green catch phrase on it, had a green lid, and had a sustainability 'certification' (the kind of certification that a company uses to certify their own products, not third party). The shampoo, of course, was full of awful stuff. But I was impressed they did such an impressive job faking being green that even he fell for it.* **❞**

Parents like Adrienne automatically trust the brand when they trust the store—and vice versa.

 ❝ *I'm fairly easy to convince if it's a product sold in Whole Foods or in that special 'natural' foods section of the regular grocery store. If it's* *sold at a gas station, I'm not buying it. No matter what the package looks like.* 99

Bonnie doesn't worry about greenwashing too much either when she shops at small natural food stores, but says she does have her guard up when she sees "natural" on products at big box and drugstores.

66 *Triclosan, sulfates, fragrance, BPA—it's hard to keep track of which ingredients to avoid and which ones are just part of internet hoaxes and speculation.* 99

Even Honey, a mother of three who lives on a small organic farm, was initially heart-warmed by a deceptively farm-friendly commercial.

66 *That Monsanto commercial of everyone round the table caught me hook, line, and sinker—until I saw the end.* 99

UL, the global independent safety science company that provides GREENGUARD and ECOLOGO certifications, offers an interactive website featuring "The Seven Sins of Greenwashing." These include hidden trade-offs, vagueness, meaningless labels, no proof, the lesser of two evils, and straight-up lying. But my personal favorite is irrelevance.

Last spring, I went to Home Depot to seek out organic seedlings for my garden. The staff directed me to a large display of non-GMO plants. Shelves full of parsley, oregano, and basil all touting non-GMO status. The problem is, there's no such thing as genetically modified herbs. These are just plain old conventional seedlings, pesticides and all.

The irrelevance borders on silliness. Toxic paint in a "recyclable" aluminum can. Oven cleaner labeled as free of a toxin that's actually been banned for 30 years. It's like labeling water as "carb and sugar free!"

But should we be rewarding companies for making small steps? When Coca-Cola offered a plant-based bottle, health and environmental advocates didn't give accolades for high-fructose corn syrup in a slightly friendlier package. Coke's Dasani water brand also now wraps itself in 30 percent plant-based material. And while that certainly doesn't make bottled water that much more sustainable, should we throw them a bone for trying?[5]

Carissa says she draws the line with products that are still inherently toxic. For her, promoting packaging progress of an unsafe product is simply greenwashing.

 66 *Ideally, we'd get all of these things: a nontoxic product packaged in a recycled/recyclable bottle, made in a LEED-certified factory with solar panels on the roofs, and free electric car chargers out front. But since there aren't too many companies that do that, I have to prioritize something. So, I prioritize toxicity of the end product.* 99

Stacy Malkan, co-founder of the Campaign for Safe Cosmetics and author of *Not Just a Pretty Face: The Ugly Side of the Beauty Industry*, agrees that we need to keep bringing the conversation back to toxicity and health.

 66 *I went to a 'sustainability summit' for the cosmetics industry and the big companies only wanted to talk about water use, recycling, and materials reductions—not the toxic chemicals they use in their products. What really sticks in my mind is Procter & Gamble saying they reduced the plastic in Gillette razors by making them lighter, thereby saving the weight equivalent of a 747 Boeing jet from going to the landfill. Now that's impressive, but I can't help thinking about how much weight in plastic is still going to the landfill every day because P&G's Gillette invented the category of disposable razors to begin with.* 99

Stacy says the same presenter from P&G went on about how the worst environmental impact of its products was the amount of water people use because they stay in the shower too long.

 66 *We have to change mindsets at a deeper level.* 99

If you want to support brands truly dedicated to doing better, Katie Holcomb, director of communications at B Lab, directs consumers to look for products certified by a disinterested third party.

❝ *It's important to not just trust advertising, but have someone actually looking at their practices. Companies need to measure their impact to track improvements and keep consumers informed.* ❞

Since 2007, B Lab has been certifying B Corporations—businesses that meet rigorous standards of social and environmental performance, accountability, and transparency. Today, there is a growing community of over 1,500 Certified B Corps from more than 40 countries and 130 industries.

Holcomb explains that a B Corporation certification looks at a company's overall impact—on its workers, its community, its consumers, and the environment.

❝ *We measure things like whether they are using renewable materials, paying their employees a living wage and hiring a diverse set of employees, and working with local communities to make them stronger.* ❞

But what if a company excels in its social mission and keeps a low-carbon footprint but still has potentially toxic chemicals in its product formulations?

❝ *We look at overall impact and embrace the idea of consistent improvement. However, it would be very difficult to meet the minimum performance requirement if you were terribly remiss in any one area. The B Impact Assessment has built-in improvement reports and best practice tools to help companies improve over time.* ❞

B Corporations have to recertify every two years, provide documentation, and are subject to a random onsite audit. My one-woman business has been certified since 2009 and audited twice, which required a guided tour of my living room.

❝ *We have a full complaints process. Anyone can make a complaint, and if it is credible and material, we send it to our standards advisory board.* ❞

But Holcomb points out that perfection is the enemy of good. Doing one unsatisfactory thing isn't necessarily going to negate you.

66 *However we do draw a line. If it's something that can't be fixed or you're not willing to fix, we determine if that requires decertification or an additional disclosure on the B Impact Report.* **99**

Taking sustainability seriously is on the radar of most large corporations as consumers grow more eco-savvy by the day. The hit-or-miss sustainability tactics of a few years ago no longer cut it with compassionate shoppers.

In recent years, various retailers have offered discounts on purchases for shoppers who use reusable bags. The only problem: some retailers required shoppers to purchase the retailer's own branded bag. This is duly irresponsible, actually encouraging needless consumption and requiring the manufacturing of thousands of problematic conventional cotton bags.

The good news is companies know we care, but we have to protect our hearts by using our heads. Ideally, there will be some new regulation on the horizon and an increase in trustworthy labeling. In the meantime, use the tips on the following page to keep you dry in a greenwashed world.

TIPS for Avoiding Greenwashing

☑ Look for authentic third-party product certifications.
These include GREENGUARD, ECOLOGO, Non-GMO
Certified, USDA Organic, B Corporation, Fair Trade USA
Certified, and Energy Star.

☑ Check out the wide variety of online shopping hubs that
specialize in eco-friendly and healthy goods. Each retailer
has its own set of standards, but they are certainly good
places to start for better products. For various needs,
visit vinemarket.com, rodales.com, thrivemarket.com,
mightynest.com, abesmarket.com, luckyvitamin.com,
and greendepot.com. And don't miss the sales and
coupon codes.

☑ Consumers can take action when they witness greenwashing by contacting corporations and policymakers to voice
concerns, or by drawing attention to misleading claims via
blogs, websites, and other outreach, according to Green-
peace's stopgreenwash.org project. You can also contact the
Federal Trade Commission or the Better Business Bureau to
register complaints.

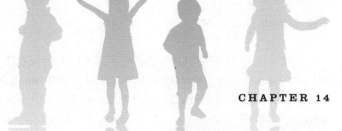

CHAPTER 14

When Best Intentions Backfire

Can Your "Green" Changes Be Less Than Eco-Friendly?

As soon as I saw a fish tank sprouting wheatgrass at my friend's house, I knew I had to have one.

I struggle to keep indoor plants alive and love having them around in the winter to improve air quality and brighten up the house. This fish tank with a garden on top works as a closed-loop ecosystem—the fish feed the plants, and the plants clean the water.

I was excited about the prospect of keeping herbs alive inside over the long, dark winter but not too thrilled about being responsible for the fragile life of a fish.

I set up the tank, and remarkably, it worked. The fish stayed alive for weeks, and the garden was resplendent with edible plants growing faster than we could consume them.

Then I checked out the roots, and they were completely covered with terrifying mold spores.

I e-mailed the company, who recommended starting over with a small fan to keep the mold spores at bay. But I wasn't going to mess around with mold. The idea was to improve air quality, not amplify our existing respiratory issues.

As sometimes happens, my attempts at living a more sustainable and healthy lifestyle had backfired. And as I write this, I am looking to see if anyone I know is in the market for a goldfish.

Sustainability, green living, healthy choices, safer products—it's all a learning curve. A curve with "curve balls" at that. Just when you think you're doing something right, you find out it's actually, well, wrong.

BPA free? Great. But we simply don't know what the BPA is being replaced with—or if it's actually worse. My babies both used BPA-free plastic bottles, so it's always fun to learn the bottles may have actually leaked their own special brand of synthetic estrogen.[1] And all those BPA-free cans? The notoriously bad plastic PVC is an FDA-approved alternative for BPA in can linings, despite the fact that vinyl chloride is a known human carcinogen.[2]

Buying vegan fur and leather? Most fake leathers are constructed from some kind of petroleum-derived plastic product. Some faux leathers are even made of PVC, a common source of phthalates.[3]

I'm not sure why you wear fur of any kind, unless you're Lil' Kim, but fake fur is made of synthetic fibers constructed from blends of acrylic and modacrylic polymers derived from coal, air, water, petroleum, and limestone. Like most plastics, fake fur also doesn't biodegrade easily.

Biodegradable dog waste bags often just create more methane gas in the landfills, so you're probably better off just repurposing your used ziplocks and random packaging.[4]

And throwing receipts in with the recycling?

Micaela Preston, blogger at mindfulmomma.com, was frustrated to learn recycled-content toilet paper was contaminated with BPA from receipt paper.[5]

    66 *I'm now very careful to never recycle receipt paper—I try to avoid taking receipts at all. But I'm on the fence about buying recycled toilet paper. Some people say it's safe, some think we should steer clear.* **99**

Personally, I still choose recycled toilet paper over virgin (and think peeing in the shower can reduce one's carbon footprint).

Recycling is probably the most common universal "green action," touted for its environmental and economic benefits.

However, an October 2015 *New York Times* opinion piece lamented our collective faith in recycling, arguing it is mostly a "feel-good" enterprise with little significant environmental or economic benefit. Writer John Tierney submits to the indisputable benefits of paper and aluminum recycling, but he debates the advantages of sorting yogurt containers and greasy pizza boxes.[6]

Richard Gertman begs to differ. Gertman, who has worked in the materials management field for more than 43 years and served as vice president of the National Recycling Coalition, says that while the economics are complicated, the environmental benefits of recycling are indisputable.

Recycling is an up-and-down venture tied to the world economy, Gertman says. By volume, the US's largest exports are scrap metal and scrap paper. Municipal programs collect these items whether or not there is a market for it, and, of course, the supply, demand, and value goes up and down.

Economics aside, though, all recycling has value. And Gertman says plastic and glass recycling hold as much benefit as paper and metal recycling.

❝ *Most plastics are produced from petroleum as a by-product, so recovering plastics allows us to use less petroleum for manufacturing. And when we use recycled glass to make new glass, we lower the temperature in the furnace, really reducing the energy required and improving the air quality.* ❞

But, Gertman says, possibly the most important advantage is one not always taken into consideration by naysayer statistics: the full cost accounting of creating a new product versus recycling something already manufactured.

❝ *If we can recycle something and not put a new product through a power plant, that's a huge difference. The alternative is to cut down more trees and mine more coal.* ❞

There are, however, some viable problems with recycling. Gertman says one of the biggest concerns is that the idea of recycling seems to give some people the liberty to consume. People may not balk at buying packages of bottled water, figuring recycling the bottles will absolve them of their consumption sins.

66 *There's the part of the equation we lose sight of. A lot of people tell me because they can recycle stuff they don't mind consuming. Ultimately, we want to reduce consumption without reducing our standard of living.* 99

Another problem is "wishcycling"—the practice of tossing questionable items in the recycling bin, hoping they can somehow be recycled.

Jen Boynton, editor in chief of triplepundit.com and mother of an 18-month-old, says she often removes plastic wrap and soiled paper from the recycling but doesn't really stress about it.

66 *With single-stream recycling, which we have in our area, there is a ton of waste that needs to get pulled out at the plant. Our missorted stuff isn't going to make a difference.* 99

But Gertman says it does make a difference—those recycling machines can't always fish your wish.

66 *Everyone wants to recycle everything they think is recyclable. People also do it to save money because, in some places, fees are charged on garbage collection but not on recyclables. In some instances, 40 percent of what is collected in recycling bins is actually garbage.* 99

Gertman says "film plastics" like plastic bags are the worst culprit, something we may intuitively *want* to recycle but which actually damage the recycling machinery.

66 *The processing equipment gets screwed up by the plastic bags, as well as anything long and stringy like Christmas lights, pants, and power cords from toasters.* 99

So no, you should not try to "wishcycle" away your torn corduroys, but the good news is you don't have to sweat the tape on Amazon packages, the grease on pizza boxes, or the specks of peanut butter stuck in the jar.

❝ *The recycling industry wants items clean because they don't want to attract pests. But in terms of the recycling, a bit of peanut butter left in the jar doesn't affect the recyclability. We grind up plastics and then we wash them because there is always residue.* ❞

In fact, Gertman says, it isn't the grease in the pizza boxes that poses a problem. It's the fact people actually try to recycle their leftover pizza.

Yes, it can be counterintuitive to use soap, water, and a paper towel to scrub a food jar clean. Gertman says it doesn't have to be spotless to be properly recycled.

❝ *Scrape out as much of the peanut butter as you can and then throw it in the bin.* ❞

Jen Boynton says the longer she works in the environmental field the more it becomes obvious there is no right and wrong—it's a spectrum.

❝ *When I make a choice, I'm weighing all kinds of factors. Sustainability and wellness are two key issues but so are price, durability, effectiveness, and convenience. There are probably 100 food decisions alone each week, and we try to be thoughtful about all of them without losing our minds.* ❞

She found cloth diapers were not the most environmental choice for her in California, where they face a massive drought. And when she tried her hand at upcycling, using old felted sweaters to make scarves as Christmas gifts, the final products were scratchy messes that fell apart due to poor sewing.

❝ *It remains a running family joke, brought up anytime I propose making something from scratch.* ❞

We aren't all meant to be homesteaders. I know that straight lines and clean corners are not my strong points. My ideas are often better than my execution, leading to a few ill-advised knitting and sewing projects of my own.

Carissa says that when she learned about the toxins in plastic, she got rid of all the plastics in her kitchen and replaced them with vintage glass ceramics.

❝ I loved the look of vintage ceramics, but then I learned that some of the old colored glass ceramic dishes have insanely high lead levels. So now we only use the clear ones. ❞

Actress Alysia Reiner used to enjoy texturized vegetable protein (TVP), a common soy by-product, as a meat substitute. This was before she became aware that the vast majority of soybeans are genetically modified and most TVP is processed with hexane, a highly explosive neurotoxic chemical.[7]

Dani Klein, comedian and author of *Afterbirth: Stories You Won't Read in a Parenting Magazine*, thought she was being proactive for her children's health by offering them gummy vitamins.

❝ I gave them to my little one for a few years, and he ended up with four cavities. It was a nightmare. Do not give gummy vitamins made with sugar to your children unless you have a family electric teeth scrubbing contest before sleeping. ❞

In an effort to be a more holistic and earth-friendly mother, I've attempted to forego chemical products and even some traditional medicine with herbal remedies, including essential oils.

After a long bout with chronic cheilitis (a fancy name for cracks in the corner of your mouth), I turned to an herbal remedy recommended by several websites: tea tree oil. I purchased a vial of the pure condensed serum and ignored the fine print about diluting the oil before use.

After applying liberally to the corners of my mouth, I tasted the strong, tingly liquid. Suddenly, I felt compelled to make sure it wouldn't be harmful to actually ingest this stuff. Thus, the dreaded Google results from mayoclinic.com: "Tea tree oil should not be used orally; there are reports of toxicity after consuming tea tree oil by mouth."

Upon absorbing these words, I completely freak out. Not only have I poisoned myself, but I will now surely poison my baby through my breast milk. I pump. I dump. I call my husband and beg him to convince me that my child and I will not die today from tea tree oil ingestion.

I faced a similar bout with the possible perils of lavender, a lovely, fragrant plant known for its relaxing properties. Widely used in aromatherapy, lavender is a common ingredient in natural baby bath and body products. Oh, and it allegedly causes baby boys to sprout Pamela Anderson-style breasts.

According to a 2007 study in the *New England Journal of Medicine*, lavender and tea tree oil contribute to gynecomastia, an abnormal breast tissue growth in prepubescent boys.[8] The author of the (albeit controversial) study writes, "The common use of products containing lavender oil, tea tree oil, or both by the three boys and the resolution of their gynecomastia within months after ceasing use of those products suggest that these oils may possess endocrine-disrupting activity that causes an imbalance in estrogen and androgen pathway signaling."

Well, that was it for lavender. I packed up all my lavender shampoos and baby calming oils and gave them to a friend with a baby girl, along with a note telling her she could thank me when she hits puberty.

Apparently, I'm not the only one who has had a snafu with natural products. Leslie Garrett, London, Ontario-based author of *The Virtuous Consumer*, says she experienced similar panic.

66 *I've had that frisson of fear upon reading about tea tree oil, which I added to kids' shampoo to prevent lice, and lavender, which I added to bath water to soothe. Fortunately, upon reading further, I learned that the teensy amounts I was using were harmless. I've also used castor oil to treat a cyst on a cat and hemp seed to help boost same cat's immune system, only to learn a week later that hemp seed can be toxic for cats because their digestive systems can't metabolize it.* 99

Information after the fact also alarmed Lisa when she learned shea butter is actually derived from a nut—something her son is allergic to.

66 I used to slather it on his lips as an alternative to petroleum-based lip balm. It never helped much, and he'd always seem to be in worse shape after I put it on. I never figured out why until my friend, an aesthetician, told me about some shea butter product she had just got at her salon and about harvesting the 'nuts from the trees.' I almost died. I had no idea I was applying a potentially deadly allergen all over my son's lips. 99

Certainly, home remedies and folk wisdom sometimes can do wonders where conventional methods fail. But, as Sarah learned, even the most benign-seeming ingredients come with their share of side effects.

66 I have a child who struggled with bedwetting for a long time. We were told the Amish give their kids honey at night. So I gave her honey and it made her so hyper she couldn't get to sleep and woke up so tired in the morning that we stopped. But she didn't wet the bed those nights! 99

And it's not just overdosing on frankincense and myrrh that has us biting our nails. (Though if you are, hot pepper and lemon juice are recommended to curb that habit.) We also face a crisis of convention when our olive oil and parsley cocktail just doesn't do the trick. We desperately want to avoid corticosteroids and antibiotics but know we have to weigh immediate relief against our long-term concerns.

Elizabeth tried natural remedies for her five-year-old's crusty ears but eventually had to give in to the hard stuff.

66 For months, I tried the organic baby lotions, which certainly help dry skin, but this seemed like something more. I didn't really want to use a steroid on her precious skin, so I resolved to find something gentler. After months, I finally I gave in and used the over-the-counter cortisone and her ears cleared up in a week. 99

Desperate to believe the answer must lie with Mother Nature, eco-conscious moms tend to beat themselves up when succumbing to traditional medicines. Personally, I believe in a mix of traditional medicine and homeopathic remedies—East meets West, acupuncture converging with acetaminophen. Essentially, my views coincide with "integrative medicine," a mix of conventional and alternative approaches, treating the whole person.

As for the "man boobs," Dr. Ronald Stram, director and founder of the Stram Center for Integrative Medicine, says the gynecomastia study was likely flawed. However, he admits that, theoretically, continued application of high doses of tea tree oil and lavender, which both have estrogenic properties, could result in such a condition. However, he says the use of these ingredients in conventional products is probably not something to worry about.

As a general rule, never use undiluted volatile oils internally, Stram says. Keep the concentration of both tea tree oil and lavender oil below 2 percent in children, and remember that too much of anything is rarely a good thing.

Home remedies can be wonderful things, and herbal medicine has many indisputable benefits. But like any good diet, the message seems to be about moderation. When in doubt, dilute. Or more preferably, ask a doctor. Or an herbalist. Or both, and let them battle it out. Just know that taking the collective temperature of your mommy message board doesn't count as an expert opinion.

When all these things that seem right are sometimes being quite wrong, it's easy to want to throw in the towel. Or we can simply try to learn from our mistakes and do better. Don't try to recycle your corduroys curbside. Try to use glass or stainless steel over plastic. Buy tomatoes that come in a jar. If you really, really want a fur coat, check out a secondhand shop near the West–Kardashian household.

T I P S for Green Choices

☑ Print and post your township's recycling guidelines. No more wishful recycling. If it can't go in the bin, it just causes more of a problem. Find recycling solutions near you at search.earth911.com

☑ Look for GMP (Good Manufacturing Practices) or USP (United States Pharmacopeia) on the label of any medicine, vitamin, homeopathic product, or dietary supplement. These official public standards-setting authorities note that the dosages listed are strictly adhered to. If a product doesn't have this label, the concentrations can vary greatly. In other words, don't buy anything from questionable sources, like unreputable websites or neighborhood witch doctors.

☑ Natural does not equal safe. Remember, tobacco and cocaine are essentially just plants.

☑ Think of concentrated oils like tequila. You know what happened the last time you drank that straight. Follow the instructions for dilution.

☑ A reasonable amount of tea tree oil and lavender in baby products probably won't cause man boobs, but I'm still sticking with aloe and calendula.

CHAPTER 15

Green Guilt:
The Jury's Verdict

Is There a Way to Ease Eco-Anxiety?

WHETHER IT'S ORGANIC vs. conventional, bottle vs. breast, or glass vs. plastic, at the center of this emotional roller coaster are millions of parents wracked with some level of guilt. Each choice is filled with anxiety, and every decision is a gateway to worry.

My own personal guilt includes but is not limited to the following: using too many paper towels, having inexplicable loyalty to Starbucks, staring at my iPhone for hours daily, and buying too many pairs of bedazzled flip-flops. And as for anxiety—well, that list would fill a whole other book.

While dealing with this internal struggle ourselves, the last thing we want is to put a sense of dread and fear into our children. After all, we make these choices so they can have better, fuller, longer lives.

But how much fun will that life be if they absorb all our negativity and neurosis?

Abby Sher, author of *Amen, Amen, Amen: Memoir of a Girl Who Couldn't Stop Praying (Among Other Things)*, says green guilt is definitely a "monster" in her home.

❝ *The books about green living usually make me excited to buy spider plants and then depressed about how little else I've done. And I can't help but wonder, is cancer so prevalent because of all these new discoveries and fragrances and cell phones?* ❞

Actress Alysia Reiner doesn't want her fretting and vigilance to create an environment of fear for her young daughter.

❝ *On a philosophical level, I don't want to believe or teach my child that the world is a dangerous place. I want my child to feel safe and happy in her world. How do you balance that out?* **❞**

The growing awareness of the 21st-century crisis has put enough people into a tizzy to yield a new form of psychology called "eco-therapy." Rebecca Elliott, MA, a life coach who specializes in "eco-anxiety," believes if parents remain present and informed, they can become part of the solution.

Elliott says we teach our children by modeling behavior. We show them by our actions how we respond to what happens in the world and give them the emotional tools to process information and respond accordingly.

When her ten-year-old son expressed concern about the possibility of a big earthquake hitting their California home, Elliott responded in a way she believes eased her child's fears.

❝ *I validated that there indeed could possibly be a large earthquake somewhere in our region. What we need to do is be aware of the possibility, take the necessary steps to have supplies on hand, and have a plan for our family in case of emergency. I assured him that our friends and neighbors in the community would come together to help each other out if anyone needed help. Until then, we keep living our lives and doing the things we love. He was completely satisfied with my explanation and didn't harbor any sense of worry about earthquakes.* **❞**

Dani Klein, comedian and author of *Afterbirth: Stories You Won't Read in a Parenting Magazine*, also mirrors her eco-anxiety lessons on the realities of earthquakes near her home in southern California.

❝ *They know about it, we take precautions, but we don't talk about it every second of every day. They actually do a great job of educating children in California about ecological issues. They come home and tell me facts about conservation they learned in school all the time. The boys* *are very aware of water conservation. They'd have to be since our shower has the pressure of a watering can.* 99

Elliott also emphasizes the importance of connecting our children with nature and allowing them to develop a loving relationship with the Earth.

66 *Children have an intrinsic love of nature. Without being told, they know how to roll down a grassy hill, make mud pies, climb trees, chase butterflies, or stare at clouds and see the shapes. Giving our kids opportunities to create indelible memories of nature is one of our highest priorities.* 99

But even as we ease our children's anxieties, we often mask our internal struggle with the fear that we don't take enough action.

Amy Wilson, actress and author of *When Did I Get Like This?*, says once in a while, her eco-anxiety leads to a great label-reading, cabinet-clearing frenzy.

66 *More often, though, I feel a low-grade guilt that I'm not doing better, but let the kids have a store-bought chocolate chip cookie anyway.* 99

Carly says she likes to think she's a good person and a positive role model for her son, but she still feels like she falls short of living up to a certain standard.

66 *I always turn the water off while I brush my teeth, and I have a reusable water bottle. However, my environmentally friendly steps seem fruitless. Everywhere I turn, I feel a sense of eco-inadequacy. I refuse to use cloth diapers. I cherish my showers too much to shorten them to five minutes. I've tried organic food shopping, but it's so expensive. I've come to terms with the fact that I'll never be the greenest mom, but I've resolved to take baby steps toward a greener lifestyle, like washing my laundry in cold water and paying all my bills online.* 99

Betsy acknowledges the difficulty in operating against the cultural norm and says she tries to do what she can and then let go as much as possible.

❝ You have to put your own sanity and your family's happiness first. I think we all have some issues we rarely bend on, but you have to pick and choose. You can't do it all. ❞

Lori says she has slowly come to terms with the fact that she can't possibly do everything to reduce her carbon footprint and remove toxins entirely from her life.

❝ I do what I can and find what fits into my family's lifestyle. I've let go of most of the guilt and focus on spreading awareness so we can all make educated decisions. ❞

Jennifer Hankey, founder of Healthy Green Schools, says the simple fact is that you can't live in a bubble and toxic chemicals are everywhere. However, does that mean we should stick our heads in the sand and ignore it because there is no point?

❝ Not at all! Even simple, small changes matter. If you make an easy change like removing artificial colors from your child's diet, that is a huge win. Get that down and then do something else—maybe high-fructose corn syrup. Over time, you will find that you have changed your whole life. It all matters. ❞

Dani Klein says sometimes she feels like it's not in our power to control things like the heat and drought issues, but she refuses to stand idly by.

❝ It will take such tremendous motivation from everyone around the world that the cynic in me questions it. But we have to at least try. We can't just throw up our hands and say, 'Bummer.' That is the most important lesson I try to teach my children every day. Do not give up—do not fall into resignation about any part of your life. Keep the faith, keep doing your part. ❞

It's tempting to want to remain in—or return to—blissful ignorance. But Zoe Weil, author of *Most Good, Least Harm*, says when the foods and products you use may ultimately harm your children and their world, that bliss can turn into even greater anxiety.

66 *Making humane and sustainable choices brings its own kind of meaning and joy and is an antidote to anxiety.* 99

Weil says that guilt isn't necessarily a bad thing.

66 *It's a sign that we have a conscious and don't want to cause harm and suffering to others. A little guilt can be the impetus for making wiser, kinder, healthier decisions, but balance is important. We should each strive to do the best we can. If we are doing that, then guilt should diminish. If we're not, then that guilt may provide the push to find that sweet spot.* 99

Weil says if we do our best to make our homes safe and work with schools and daycare centers to do the same, then our children will by and large be protected.

66 *Then we need to let go and let our kids just be kids. There is a growing fear of what may happen to them outdoors—ticks and Lyme disease, mosquitoes and Eastern equine encephalitis, sunshine and skin cancer—yet 'protecting' our children from the outdoors is terrible. The natural world is our true home, the source of deep connection, reverence, wonder, awe, and beauty. Additionally, if we don't love the Earth, we have less incentive to protect it, which is the real peril our children face.* 99

Rebecca Elliott recognized the mind-boggling task of trying to keep up with the tremendous change occurring in the world, but to keep our sanity, she says we can do a few things.

66 *Believe in yourself, trust your instincts, and stick to what you're committed to. Acknowledge and applaud the efforts that you have made, whether they are big or small. Know that one change leads to another, and over time you'll begin to notice how much of your day-to-day life is more sustainable.* 99

Elliott also emphasizes the benefits of simplicity and the importance of accepting our shortcomings.

❝ *Sustainability and simplicity do not have to be about deprivation. Living a more simplistic lifestyle can actually become more freeing. In the quest to be perfect parents in this age of environmental information overload, we're bound to make mistakes. At the end of the day, we're still human and can only do so much. We need to make sure we give ourselves permission to not be perfect, to not be so hard on ourselves, and to be OK with doing what we can while letting the rest go.* ❞

Jen Pleasants, author of *Bag Green Guilt, Five Easy Steps: Turn Eco-Anxiety Into Constructive Energy*, has also explored eco-anxiety and green guilt as common by-products from the pressure to be green. She says we need to learn how to funnel those feelings into constructive channels and feel reassured that what we do *does* make a difference.

As a stressed out mother of three, Pleasants found solace through the tips in her book and considers herself a more productive and happier member of society.

❝ *I was able to get out of my fetal position, stop feeling so overwhelmed, and start making steps for a healthier self and Earth.* ❞

Fortunately, for those moments where we wallow in futility and sorrow, planet cheerleaders like Michele Beschen, host of *b. organic with Michele Beschen* on PBS, help clarify the silver lining among the clouds of doom and gloom.

❝ *I still see a beautiful planet that is filled with resourceful, innovative, caring people—people who every day are becoming more in tune to the environment and healthy living. I only see those efforts growing and evolving further in the right direction.* ❞

Betsy believes pessimism about the environment and the future in general can harm children, so she tries to emphasize the good.

❝ *Kids are surrounded with environmental bad news, so I try hard to highlight the positive—people making a difference, success stories, and humanity's efforts to try to fix our mistakes.* **❞**

Elliott also emphasizes the growing sense of community due to awareness of the environmental devastation.

❝ *Hundreds of thousands of people globally are joining forces and mobilizing efforts to enact positive change in environmental and social justice.* **❞**

Weil believes we create a better world by providing young people with the knowledge, tools, and motivation to be solutionaries for a just, humane, and sustainable future.

Through this sense of community and possibility, it becomes plausible to see the glass as half full. The growing awareness of a planet in peril has literally made us stop and smell the roses. Suddenly, we all know what Joni Mitchell was talking about when she said, "They paved paradise and put up a parking lot."

The world may be getting warmer, but the good news is the next generation is getting smarter. Cigarettes could be obsolete in 50 years, and our kids now teach us how to compost.

I am not perfect, nor are my children. I am guilty of using food as a reward, making separate dinners consisting entirely of carbs, allowing too much screen time, and letting my children believe no dinner is complete without dessert.

But, yes, I believe I am making a difference. Despite loving a Hershey bar as much as the next kid, my son *gets it.*

He understands the difference between "healthy food" and "junky food" and knows that too much sugar will make his belly hurt. He doesn't run like Pavlov's dog at the sound of an ice cream truck. He prides himself on choosing the less offensive pretzels when offered a choice of prepackaged cookies at camp. He realizes cheap toys will break immediately and thinks it's cool we make our own healthy piñatas and Easter egg hunts.

The green movement has been more than a call to arms to protect the planet, question consumerism, and take stock of our health. The backlash against materialism has brought a return to simplicity, offering a welcome respite from our multitasking smartphones as we make time to embrace growing our own basil and hemming our own skirts.

For all its intentions to offer "better living through chemistry" and information superhighways, the new world we live in takes a lot more than a GPS to navigate. But the plus side is that information is power, and while the choices aren't simple, at least we have the knowledge to make better—if not perfect—decisions.

Actress Kaitlin Olson says with a little research and planning, it's not terribly difficult to find great safe options for food, home, and personal care products.

66 *So far, my kids don't feel like they are missing out on anything. I want them to enjoy life! I'm just trying to teach them how to make healthy choices to keep their bodies strong and safe. I don't try to scare them into doing it by pointing out how dangerous everything is. I save that for their poor teachers.* 99

And as safer, cleaner products and sustainable living become more mainstream, it will be that much easier for our children to make good choices without a second thought.

Dad Ryan notes that his children won't know a world where you couldn't find a single organic item in a big box store.

66 *As children, we were ingrained to think these conventional brands were trusted companies, but our kids are going to know that these organic brands are what we use.* 99

We can also fight for our right to better information, honesty from manufacturers, and stricter standards from the government. Remember, irate moms in Canada helped enforce BPA legislation. Grassroots consumer efforts got artificial dyes removed from macaroni and cheese, and brominated vegetable oil (patented as a flame retardant and banned in Europe and Japan) out of Gatorade. It was the efforts of one mother, Leah Segedie, that pushed the American Academy of Pediatrics to break ties with Monsanto.

And even as I do the final proof of these pages, change is happening faster than I can type.

In 2014, Vermont became the first state to make GMO labeling mandatory. And, in response, House Representatives passed federal legislation to preempt states from requiring the labeling of GMO foods. This legislation became known in the consumer rights community as the "Deny Americans the Right-to-Know (DARK) Act." But, in March 2016, the DARK Act failed to pass in the Senate. While labeling advocates were hopeful but cautious, seeing this as a temporary reprieve, the weeks immediately following were vastly significant.

Within days, General Mills made the announcement that it would begin labeling all genetically modified foods. They were following in the footprints of Campbell's, who had made a similar announcement in January. And then the dominos began rapidly falling—Kellogg's, Mars, ConAgra, Del Monte. Announcements of large corporations labeling GMOs are beginning to snowball.

Robyn O'Brien said we should let Annie's be the compass for General Mills, and her optimism rang true. Change was being sparked from inside, stoked by the fires of a million consumer voices.

In no small part this change has been driven by the passing of Vermont's law. Large food companies realized that once the Vermont law is enacted in July 2016, it would be nearly impossible to craft new labels for each state. Companies also likely concluded that it would be cheaper and easier to simply apply the new label to all of their products, thus making little Vermont's law the *de facto* national standard.[1]

Knowledge will evolve, but we can hold fast to certain eternal truths. Swallowed gum won't stay in your stomach for seven years, potatoes will not grow behind dirty ears, and if your kids keep making that face, it won't freeze and stay that way forever.

As for everything else—as we know better, we can do better. Not always best, certainly not perfect, but better.

TIPS for Assuaging Green Guilt

☑ Work to enact political change that will make a difference on a larger scale. Vote for candidates with strong environmental initiatives. Write letters and send e-mails, from complaints about your school district's lack of recycling to petitions to the federal government. Get things off your chest and use your voice to feel empowered.

☑ Get outdoors with your children and instill an appreciation of nature.

☑ Lead by example. We can't control the world around us, but we can control what we do in our own space.

☑ Pat yourself on the back. Remember that perfect is an unattainable goal, and everything you can do makes a difference.

Notes

Foreword

1. See "Toxic Chemicals," nrdc.org/issues/toxic-chemicals.
2. See WHO Fact Sheet no. 292, "Household air pollution and health," who.int/mediacentre/factsheets/fs292/en/, and Fact Sheet no. 352, "Environmental and occupational cancers," who.int/mediacentre /factsheets/fs350/en/.
3. See "Bill Gates Q&A on Climate Change: 'We Need a Miracle'," Bloomberg News, 22 Feb 2016, bloomberg.com/news/articles/2016 -02-23/bill-gates-q-a-on-climate-change-we-need-a-miracle.

Chapter 1

1. Shallow, Parvati. "Kraft Removing Artificial Dyes, Preservatives from Mac & Cheese." CBS News. CBS Interactive, 20 Apr 2015.
2. "T-BUTYLHYDROQUINONE." U.S. National Library of Medicine: Toxicology Data Network, n.d. Web. 11 Dec 2015.
3. Hamblin, James. "The Dark Side of Almond Use." *The Atlantic*, 28 Aug 2014. Web. 28 Nov 2015.

Chapter 2

1. Strom, Stephanie. "Cereals Begin to Lose Their Snap, Crackle and Pop." *The New York Times*, 10 Sept 2014.
2. DePillis, Lydia. "Is America over Soup?" *The Washington Post*, 20 Nov 2013. Web. 28 Nov 2015.
3. Nicolaou, Anna. "McDonald's Sees Drop in Customers as Scandals Start to Bite." *Financial Times*. n.p., 22 Apr 2015. Web. 28 Nov 2015.
4. "IWF Issues: Culture of Alarmism." IWF Issues. Web. 16 Dec 2015. iwf.org/culture-of-alarmism.
5. "10 Companies That Control the World's Food." MarketWatch. n.p., 2 Sept 2014. marketwatch.com/story/10-companies-that-control-the -worlds-food-2014-09-01.
6. CommonGround, organizational website homepage, Web. Dec 2015.

7. "CommonGround." SourceWatch. Web. 16 Dec 2015. sourcewatch.org /index.php/commonground.

8. Halzack, Sarah. "Your Healthy Habits Are Eating into the Packaged Foods Industry." *The Washington Post*, 13 Feb 2015.

9. Jarvis, Rebecca, and Susanna Kim. "General Mills to Eliminate Artificial Colors, Flavors From Entire Cereal Line." ABC News, 22 June 2015.

10. Malcolm, Hadley. "Taco Bell, Pizza Hut Nix Artificial Ingredients." *USA Today*, 26 May 2015.

11. Aubrey, Allison. "Panera Is The Latest To Drop Artificial Ingredients From Its Food." NPR, 6 May 2015.

12. Landau, Elizabeth. "Subway to Remove Chemical from Bread - CNN .com." CNN. Cable News Network, 17 Feb 2014.

13. Peterson, Hayley. "McDonald's Is Rolling out Its First Organic Hamburger and It Looks Amazing." *Business Insider*, 25 Sept 2015.

Chapter 3

1. Lehrburger, Carl. *Diapers in the Waste Stream: A Review of Waste Management and Public Policy Issues*. Sheffield, MA: self-published, 1989.

2. Little, Arthur D. *Disposable Versus Reusable Diapers: Health, Environmental and Economic Comparisons: Report to Procter and Gamble, March 16, 1990*. Cambridge, MT: Arthur D. Little, Inc., 1990.

3. Aumônier, Simon, Michael Collins, and Peter Garrett. *An Updated Lifecycle Assessment Study for Disposable and Reusable Nappies*. The Environment Agency, Bristol, UK, 1990. Web.

Chapter 4

1. Sears, Bill. "Taking Medications Safely While Breastfeeding." askdr .sears.com. Web. 5 Oct 2015. askdrsears.com/topics/feeding-eating/ breastfeeding/while-taking-medication/taking-medications-safely -while-breastfeeding/weigh.

2. Hale, Ph.D., T.W. Dr. Hale's Breastfeeding and Medications Forum. Texas Tech University Health Sciences Center School of Medicine at Amarillo, n.d. Web. 5 Oct 2015. infantrisk.com/forum/forum.

3. Williams, Florence. "Toxic Breast Milk?" *The New York Times*, 9 Jan 2005.

Chapter 5

1. Sweeny, Glynis. "Fast Fashion Is the Second Dirtiest Industry in the World, Next to Big Oil." EcoWatch. n.p., 17 Aug 2015.

Chapter 6

1. "Senate Passes Final Reform Bill – Headed to President's Desk." Safer Chemicals, Healthy Families, 20 June 2016. http://saferchemicals.org/newsroom/senate-passes-final-reform-bill-headed-to-presidents-desk/

2. "Multi-State Survey of Dollar Store Products." The Ecology Center, 4 Feb 2015. Web.

Chapter 7

1. Stein, Rob. "Millions of H1N1 vaccine doses may have to be discarded." *The Washington Post*, 1 Apr 2010.

2. Brody, Jane E. "Babies Know: A Little Dirt Is Good for You." *The New York Times*, 26 Jan 2009.

3. Strachan, D. P. "Hay fever, Hygiene, and Household Size." *British Medical Journal*. 299, 1989.

4. "Asthma: The Hygiene Hypothesis." U.S. Department of Health and Human Services. FDA U.S. Food and Drug Administration, 18 Jun 2009. Web.

5. Thomas, Katie. "The 'No More Tears' Shampoo, Now With No Formaldehyde." *The New York Times*, 17 Jan 2014.

6. Mayaud, L., A. Carricajo, A. Zhiri, and G. Aubert. "Comparison of Bacteriostatic and Bactericidal Activity of 13 Essential Oils against Strains with Varying Sensitivity to Antibiotics." Letters in Applied Microbiology. The Society for Applied Microbiology, 22 Aug 2008.

Chapter 8

1. Aleccia, JoNel. "Kitchen Calamity: Reports of Shattering Cookware on the Rise." today.com. n.p., 21 Dec 2012. today.com/health/kitchen-calamity-reports-shattering-cookware-rise-1C7700507.

2. "Keurig Recalling Nearly 7 Million Coffee Makers—NBC News." NBC News. n.p., 23 Dec 2014.

3. "Teflon and Other Non-stick Pans Kill Birds." EWG. n.p., 3 Apr 2003. ewg.org/research/pfcs-global-contaminants/teflon-and-other-non-stick-pans-kill-birds.

4. Suja, Fatihah, Biplob Kumar Pramanik, and Shahrom Md. Zain. "Contamination, Bioaccumulation and Toxic Effects of Perfluorinated Chemicals (PFCs) in the Water Environment: A Review Paper." Water Science & Technology 60(6): 1533, 2009. Web. niehs.nih.gov/health/materials/perflourinated_chemicals_508.pdf.

5. "Bisphenol A." National Toxicology Program. National Institute of

Environmental Health Sciences. n.p., n.d. Web. 30 Oct 2015.
niehs.nih.gov/health/assets/docs_a_e/bisphenol_a_bpa_508.pdf.

6. Yang, C. Z., S. I. Yaniger, V. C. Jordan, D. J. Klein, and G. D. Bittner.
"Most Plastic Products Release Estrogenic Chemicals: A Potential
Health Problem That Can Be Solved. " *Environmental Health Per-*
spectives. 119:989–96. 2 March 2011. ncbi.nlm.nih.gov/pubmed
/21367689.

7. Gross, Liza. "Flame Retardants in Consumer Products Are Linked to
Health and Cognitive Problems." *The Washington Post*, 15 April 2013.

8. Olsen G. W, J. M. Burris, D. J. Ehresman, J. W. Froehlich, A. M. Seacat,
J. L. Butenhoff, and L. R. Zobel. "Half-life of serum elimination of per-
fluorooctanesulfonate, perfluorohexanesulfonate and perfluoroocta-
noate in retired fluorochemical production workers." Environmental
Health Perspectives 115:1298–1305, 2007.

Chapter 9

1. Hamblin, James. "The Ingredient to Avoid in Soap." *The Atlantic*,
17 Nov 2014. theatlantic.com/health/archive/2014/11/forget-anti
bacterial-products/382832/.

2. "FDA Taking Closer Look at 'Antibacterial' Soap." U.S. Food and
Drug Administration, 16 Dec 2013. Web. 6 Dec 2015. fda.gov/for
consumers/consumerupdates/ucm378393.htm.

3. ."Hall of Shame | EWG's 2015 Guide to Sunscreens." Hall of Shame |
EWG's 2015 Guide to Sunscreens. Web. 8 Feb 2016.

Chapter 10

1. Jones Putnam, Judith, and J. E. Allshouse. "Food Consumption, Prices,
and Expenditures, 1970–97." United States Department of Agriculture,
Economic Research Service, n.d.

2. Barclay, Eliza. "Your Grandparents Spent More Of Their Money On
Food Than You Do." NPR, 2 Mar 2015.

3. Clauson, Annette. "Despite Higher Food Prices, Percent of U.S. Income
Spent on Food Remains Constant." United States Department of
Agriculture, Economic Research Service, Sep 2008.

4. Hill, Graham. "Living With Less. A Lot Less." *The New York Times*, 9
Mar 2013.

Chapter 11

1. "Trouble in Toyland." U.S. PIRG Education Fund, Nov 2013. Web.

uspirgedfund.org/sites/pirg/files/reports/usp%20toyland%202013
%201.3.pdf.

2. Bock, Kenneth. *Healing the New Childhood Epidemics: Autism, ADHD,
   Asthma, and Allergies: The Groundbreaking Program for the 4-A Disor-
   ders*. New York: Ballantine, 2008.

3. "Cancer in Children and Adolescents." National Cancer Institute.
   Web. 27 Oct 2015. cancer.gov/types/childhood-cancers/child
   -adolescent-cancers-fact-sheet.

Chapter 12

1. Rosenthal, Elisabeth. "Your Biggest Carbon Sin May Be Air Travel."
   The New York Times, 26 Jan 2013. Web. 27 Oct 2015.

2. Jones, Charisse. "Air Travel Demand Projected to Double in 20 Years."
   USA Today. Gannett, 8 June 2015. Web. 27 Oct 2015.

Chapter 13

1. Kaufman, Leslie. "Mr. Whipple Left It Out: Soft Is Rough on Forests."
   The New York Times, 25 Feb 2009. Web. 11 Dec 2015.

2. "Cascade Dishwasher Detergent Gel." EWG's Guide to Healthy Cleaning, n.d. Web. ewg.org/guides/cleaners/1604-cascadedishwasher
   detergentgel.

3. "Kleenex® Bathroom Hand Towels Product Details| Kleenex® Brand."
   kleenex.com. n.p., n.d. Web. 11 Dec 2015. kleenex.com/handtowels
   detail.aspx.

4. "Lysol Professional Disinfectant Spray, Crisp Linen Cleaner Rating."
   EWG's Guide to Healthy Cleaning. n.p., n.d. Web. 11 Dec 2015.
   ewg.org/guides/cleaners/1204-lysolprofessionaldisinfectantspray
   crisplinen.

5. "PlantBottle Frequently Asked Questions." The Coca-Cola Company.
   n.p., n.d. Web. 11 Dec 2015. coca-colacompany.com/stories/plant
   bottle-frequently-asked-questions/.

Chapter 14

1. Bilbrey, Jenna. "BPA-Free Plastic Containers May Be Just as Hazard-
   ous." *Scientific American*, 11 Aug 2014. Web.

2. "FAQ: BPA and Alternatives." *FAQ: BPA and Alternatives*. Breast Cancer
   Fund, n.d. Web. 27 Oct 2015.

3. Sheppard, Kate. "Is Fake Leather Really More Eco-Friendly Than
   Real?" *Mother Jones*. n.p., 24 Jan 2011. Web. 11 Dec 2015.

4. Gilson, Dave. "Do Biodegradable Plastics Really Work?" *Mother Jones*. n.p., May–Jun 2009. Web. 11 Dec 2015.
5. Nuwer, Rachel. "Check Your Receipt: It May Be Tainted." Green Blog. *The New York Times*, 1 Nov 2011.
6. Tierney, John. "The Reign of Recycling." *The New York Times*, 3 Oct 2015.
7. "Behind the Bean: The Heroes and Charlatans of the Natural and Organic Soy Foods Industry." The Cornucopia Institute. n. p., 2009. Web.
8. Henley, D.V., K.S. Korach, N. Lipson, and C.A. Bloch. "Prepubertal gynecomastia linked to lavender and tea tree oils." *New England Journal of Medicine* 356. 2007.

Chapter 15
1. Hopkinson, Jenny. "How Vermont Beat Big Food." *Politico*. Web. 27 Mar 2016.

Resources

A list of suggested and referenced books, websites, and businesses

Food
thrivemarket.com
luckyvitamin.com
vitacost.com

localharvest.org
hungryharvest.net

Diapers
realdiaperassociation.org

clothdiapertrader.com

Milk
kellymom.com
mommymeds.com

infantrisk.com

Clothing
poshmark.com
thredup.com

totspot.com
yerdle.com

My comprehensive list of affordable, sustainable fashion brands at
spitthatoutthebook.com/2012/10/updated-list-eco-fashion-brands/

Toys
healthytoys.org
rosiehippo.com
mamamayishop.com

oompa.com
thesoftlanding.com

Health and Beauty
nomoredirtylooks.com
kind-eye.com
ewg.org/skindeep
nontoxiccertified.org

safecosmetics.org

Home

naturepedic.com

mightynest.com

abesmarket.com

globalgirlfriend.com

vivaterra.com

greenheartshop.org

bambeco.com

School

thelunchtray.com

healthygreenschools.com

greenschoolsalliance.org

centerforgreenschools.org

recyclebank.com

Money and Sharing Economy

biggreenpurse.com

buynothingproject.org

sharingisgoodbook.com

Coupons and Deal Sites

ebates.com

mambosprouts.com

organicdeals.com

recyclebank.com

thegreenbacksgal.com

wholefoodsmarket.com/coupons

berrycart.com

jet.com and zulily.com are both online marketplaces with deep savings on all sorts of products, including some great eco-friendly brands. Just be aware that both do drop shipping, which means an order may come in several different packages, which can be wasteful in itself.

Travel

greenloons.com

carbonfootprint.com

Advocacy and Activism

change.org

momsrising.org

organicconsumers.org

saferchemicals.org

womensvoices.org

momscleanairforce.org

healthychild.org

ewg.org

earthjustice.org

foodandwaterwatch.org

mamavation.com

fooddemocracynow.org

endfoodwastenow.org

Films Worth Watching

MisLEAD: The Movie

Toxic Baby

Unacceptable Levels

Food Inc.

Fed Up
Gasland (1 and 2)
Toxic Hotseat
The Human Experiment

Consumed
The Kids Menu
Stink!

Books Worth Reading

Animal, Vegetable, Miracle: A Year of Food Life by Barbara Kingsolver. New York: Harper Perennial, 2008.

Big Green Purse: Use Your Spending Power to Create a Cleaner, Greener World by Diane McEachern. New York: Avery, 2008.

Eat Pretty: Nutrition for Beauty, Inside and Out by Jolene Hart. San Francisco: Chronicle Books, 2014.

An Inconvenient Truth: The Crisis of Global Warming by Al Gore. New York: Viking Books for Young Readers, 2007.

In Defense of Food: An Eater's Manifesto by Michael Pollan. New York: Penguin Books, 2009.

Magnifeco: Your Head-to-Toe Guide to Ethical Fashion and Non-Toxic Beauty by Kate Black. Gabriola Island, BC: New Society Publishers, 2015.

Most Good, Least Harm: A Simple Principle for a Better World and Meaningful Life by Zoe Weil. New York: Atria Books/Beyond Words, 2009.

No More Dirty Looks: The Truth about Your Beauty Products—and the Ultimate Guide to Safe and Clean Cosmetics by Siobhan O'Connor and Alexandra Spunt. New York: Da Capo Lifelong Books, 2010.

Not Just a Pretty Face: The Ugly Side of the Beauty Industry by Stacy Malkan. Gabriola Island, BC: New Society Publishers, 2007.

The Omnivore's Dilemma: A Natural History of Four Meals by Michael Pollan. New York: Penguin, 2007.

Plastic-Free: How I Kicked the Plastic Habit and How You Can Too by Beth Terry. New York: Skyhorse Publishing, 2015.

Raising Baby Green: The Earth-Friendly Guide to Pregnancy, Childbirth, and Baby Care by Dr. Alan Greene. New York: Jossey-Bass, 2007.

Raising Elijah: Protecting Our Children in an Age of Environmental Crisis by Sandra Steingraber. New York: Da Capo Press, 2013.

Slow Death by Rubber Duck: The Secret Danger of Everyday Things by Rick Smith and Bruce Lourie. Berkeley, CA: Counterpoint, 2010.

Smart Mama's Green Guide: Simple Steps to Reduce Your Child's Toxic Chemical Exposure by Jennifer Taggart. New York: Center Street, 2009.

This Changes Everything: Capitalism vs. The Climate by Naomi Klein. New York: Simon & Schuster, 2015.

Toxin Toxout: Getting Harmful Chemicals Out of Our Bodies and Our World by Bruce Lourie and Rick Smith. New York: St. Martin's Press, 2014.

The Unhealthy Truth: One Mother's Shocking Investigation into the Dangers of America's Food Supply—and What Every Family Can Do to Protect Itself by Robyn O'Brien. New York: Harmony, 2010.
Unjunk Your Junk Food: Healthy Alternatives to Conventional Snacks by Andrea Donsky. New York: Gallery Books, 2011.

Additional Sources and Contributors

humaneeducation.org

robynobrien.com

kiwimagonline.com

storyofstuff.com

triplepundit.com

bcorporation.net

drgreene.com

mommygreenest.com

mamavation.com

mindfulmomma.com

groovygreenlivin.com

wereparentsblog.com

eco-novice.com

green-talk.com

living-consciously.com

embracingimperfect.com

creativegreenliving.com

Acknowledgments

First and foremost, this book would not have been possible without the generous contributions of personal stories from my "parents' sounding board." Thank you to each and every one of you for your time and your honesty.

I am abundantly thankful for the help and support of my husband, editor, and best friend Mike Bederka.

Thank you to my parents for your support and infinite supply of story material.

Thank you to Chris Tomasino for believing in this project—for the almost six years it took to get it published.

Thank you, Beth Buczynski, for showing the true meaning of "sharing." And to New Society Publishers for helping me share these stories far and wide.

To all the "Warriors" and "Changemakers" who know who they are—what we are building together is revolutionary and real.

Index

About the Author

PAIGE WOLF is a publicist, author, advocate, and eco-chic living expert. Paige regularly appears as a green living expert on television, in print, and at conferences across the country. A widely read author, she's received national acclaim from *people.com*, *Pregnancy & Newborn Magazine*, *Babble*, and more. Paige lives in Philadelphia with her husband and two children, where she runs Paige Wolf Media & Public Relations, a Certified B Corporation offering communications services to clients who contribute to a sustainable world and positive change. To learn more, visit spitthatoutthebook.com and paigewolf.com.

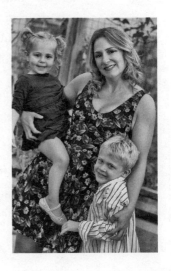

If you have enjoyed *Spit That Out!*, you might also enjoy other

BOOKS TO BUILD A NEW SOCIETY

Our books provide positive solutions for people who
want to make a difference. We specialize in:

Climate Change ◆ Conscious Community
Conservation & Ecology ◆ Cultural Critique
Education & Parenting ◆ Energy ◆ Food & Gardening
Health & Wellness ◆ Modern Homesteading & Farming
New Economies ◆ Progressive Leadership ◆ Resilience
Social Responsibility ◆ Sustainable Building & Design

New Society Publishers
ENVIRONMENTAL BENEFITS STATEMENT

New Society Publishers has chosen to produce this book on recycled paper made
with 100% post consumer waste, processed chlorine free, and old growth free.

For every 5,000 books printed, New Society saves the following resources:[1]

20	Trees
1,772	Pounds of Solid Waste
1,949	Gallons of Water
2,543	Kilowatt Hours of Electricity
3,221	Pounds of Greenhouse Gases
14	Pounds of HAPs, VOCs, and AOX Combined
5	Cubic Yards of Landfill Space

---

[1]Environmental benefits are calculated based on research done by the Environmental Defense Fund and
other members of the Paper Task Force who study the environmental impacts of the paper industry.

For a full list of NSP's titles, please call 1-800-567-6772 or check out our web site at:

www.newsociety.com

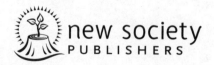
new society PUBLISHERS